DEFEATIN

DEFEATING DYSLEXIA

A Boy's Story

PARIS INNES

KYLE CATHIE LIMITED

First published 1990 by
Kyle Cathie Limited
3 Vincent Square London SW1P 2LX

ISBN 1 85626 006 2

A Cataloguing in Publication record for this title
is available from the British Library.

Typeset by DP Photosetting, Aylesbury, Bucks
Printed and bound in Great Britain by
Cox & Wyman Ltd., Reading, Berks.

To Mum and Dad,
for making this possible

CONTENTS

INTRODUCTION

by SUSAN HAMPSHIRE

Dyslexia was medically recognised in 1975 and since then hardly a week has gone by when I have not been involved in some way in increasing awareness of this handicap, not least by writing two books to raise money for the cause (*Susan's Story* – mine! and *Every Letter Counts* – success stories of famous and not so famous dyslexics).

My passionate concern for my fellow sufferers is not because I am dyslexic myself. I have been one of the lucky ones whose family support, coupled with my own determination, has pulled me through. But knowing that there are so many dyslexics who still need help leaves me with a constant nagging concern that still not enough is being done. Until there is specialist help for all sufferers, books such as *Defeating Dyslexia* which give encouragement are very important.

There are about two million dyslexics in Britain, thousands of whom have never been assessed, given specialist help or even had family support. This includes many of the 350,000 dyslexic schoolchildren whose difficulty may not have been picked up. Many have been wrongly diagnosed as lazy, stupid or retarded, and misdirected into remand homes, mental hospitals or schools catering for children with emotional problems, when their main need is specialist teaching.

If you break your arm or twist your ankle, people can see your difficulty and help you. But as dyslexia is not visible, many people are confused by it and are not sure *how* to help. So it is a tremendous joy to me to see the achievements of a young dyslexic like Paris who, with the help of his computer, has written this lively book.

Although a word processor can be very helpful, a computer may not be the answer to every dyslexic's difficulties, and I hasten to say it would be foolhardy for parents to rush out and buy one without first thoroughly examining their child's needs. Nevertheless, Paris and his computer are proof that there are more ways than one to come to terms with this hidden handicap. I am sure this book will inspire dyslexics and parents alike to persevere and explore every available avenue so that the dyslexic sufferer can achieve his or her full potential.

Susan Hampshire

FOREWORD

The purpose of this book is threefold. Firstly, it gives our 14-year-old son, Paris, the chance to describe what it is like to be dyslexic, and what he has had to do in order to overcome it.

Secondly, Paris has the opportunity to display his short stories. He wrote these on a word processor, mostly in the course of the daily sessions he went through in order to learn how to use the machine and all its functions. Writing the stories gave him the incentive to persist, and it is learning to use this word processor that has made such an enormous difference to his ability to communicate.

Finally, the book shows our experiences as the parents of a dyslexic child, the problems we have had to face and the solutions we have found.

Paris is not a child genius, nor is he outstandingly gifted. He is a happy, well adjusted 14-year-old who until recently has been performing 40–50% below his ability because he suffers from dyslexia. This book should be read in that context, although it does not stop his stories being entertaining.

Just over a year ago, after seven years at school, Paris's writing was barely legible, he misspelled or misused 20–25% of the words he wrote, and he never wrote a story much over a hundred words. Now he can write a story of over 600 words in half an hour, with a one per cent error rate.

Many parents may feel they do not have the time or the patience to teach their child to type or use a word processor. Mastering it took between 25 and 30 hours, at the rate of an hour a night. It took persistence, but at least it shows what can be done.

We have written our section of the book from our own experiences, as parents. We hope that other parents – or children or adults faced with the problems of dyslexia – will find our experiences of some help.

Trevor and Maggie Innes
May 1990

WHAT HAVING DYSLEXIA HAS MEANT TO ME

by PARIS INNES

When I was twelve I used to cry in my bed at night and tell my Mum that I wished I was normal. My Mum said that I was good at sport and had lots of things going for me. I told her I wished I wasn't good at any of those things, I just wanted to be able to read and write properly.

Before I was aware that I had dyslexia everyone told me that I was average. Even when I found out I was dyslexic, and the teachers also knew, they still said I was fine, but the fact is that I wasn't. There was no positive criticism because I think they don't really know what to do or how to help children with learning difficulties like dyslexia.

When we found out that I was dyslexic, I felt a total failure, that I was no good to anyone, and that I would end up on the street with no home and no family. I even tried to run away from home, but I only got as far as the end of the street because my bags were too heavy and my Dad came and got me.

In class I felt really stupid and didn't like my handwriting. When everyone else's handwriting was getting better, mine if anything seemed to get worse. It was always a task to read and write, so I didn't do this unless I had to.

When I started to go to the Dyslexic Centre for extra lessons twice a week, I felt different from everyone else, which I hated. It was costing my parents £23 per week and that made me feel bad because it wasn't really helping me much, and my writing was no better. Using the book *Alpha to Omega*, which is aimed at dyslexics, did help me a little in the spelling of words. It was the first time I had been taught how to sound out the words phonetically, which was much better than the 'Look and Learn' method with which I was taught in primary school. At my primary school I also received remedial teaching, especially in reading. I still hate to read much, so obviously it didn't do me a lot of good.

At secondary school I received extra teaching as well but it still didn't help. At the lessons we just reviewed everything that we had done in primary school and I wasn't catching up with the other kids in my class.

My family have a friend who is very dyslexic. He is a doctor (a very good one at that, because he is now a leading authority on asthma and lectures around the world), and he found his problem was helped when he bought a Sinclair Spectrum home computer. Typing made it much easier for him to read what he had written, and helped him a lot with his work. He's written a piece for this book about what *he* feels about being dyslexic.

My Dad bought a secondhand Amstrad 8256 computer. I learnt to touch type and I started to write stories but there was one snag – it wasn't helping with my spelling. After much searching and research we got in touch with Smith Corona and they sold us a word processor with a 'Spell-Right' dictionary and a 'Word-Right' Autospell, which bleeps at you when you spell a word wrong, and allows you to replace an incorrect word by touching a key.

I became more confident and as I wrote more stories, I felt better, knowing that I was able to spell and write neatly. Before I had the word processor, I wrote a few stories for school but they were terrible because you could not read them. I used to say that it didn't matter, because *I* could read them and that was what counted.

When I am on my word processor and it bleeps to say that I have spelt a word wrong, I feel livid, but when the spelling comes up and it's corrected I feel better again. If I spell a word wrong I may not know if it is right or wrong. The best thing about the 'Spell-Right' dictionary is that it checks my spelling much faster than if I looked up a word in an ordinary dictionary.

I hate editing my work, because everyone always says that it is fine, apart from the mistakes. But how can it be fine if it has mistakes?

When we bought the word processor I had to do an hour's work every day over the Christmas holidays, except Christmas Day. This was so that I would be ready to take it to school to do my work on at the start of term in January 1989. At first I hated it, and would get angry with my Dad for making me work all the time. I would cry myself to sleep at night, which my Mum and Dad don't know about, but I soon got used to it, and I am now very strict with myself and do some homework even if I do not have any from school.

I once wrote a story that was called *The House on the Hill* about the rivalry between Tesco's and Sainsbury's. The people in the original story had different names, which could not be used in a children's book. My Dad didn't know until we edited the stories for my book that I was secretly calling him a *******, because I was angry at him for making me write a story every night. This happened when I had first got the word processor.

The most important thing is I have learnt the real skill of typing, which has helped me a lot in writing my stories. But it did not stop there. Since I learnt how to use the Smith Corona PWP I have gone on to learn about more advanced computers and programs, so I have a constant challenge learning.

I am not trying to say it's a miracle cure, because it is not! You have to work constantly, and keep going no matter what. Dyslexia will not go away overnight, but the word processor will give you skills that will help you in later life. I think my word processor is the best thing that has ever happened to me and I would recommend it to any one.

I have mainly thought of the ideas for my stories through TV. As I couldn't read very well, TV kept my mind working and thinking. I am not saying that you should watch TV all the time, but it helped me.

I wish I had been able to read more and write properly, because it is a gift that most people take for granted, and they don't understand why I can't do it. Many of my friends have this gift and they are just throwing it away.

When I try to read, it is as if the book was written in a foreign language. I have to translate every word into 'dyslexic' so that I can understand what the words are saying. When I was reading out loud to my class or in public, I always felt embarrassed in case I got it wrong, and people would think I was stupid.

Reading has always been a great problem for me, and I have never been able to understand why, when it comes naturally to everyone else. If I read a normal book, I have to concentrate so hard on reading each word, to figure out what it is, I then cannot understand what the sentence is I have just read. This makes me read very slowly, and then most of the time I still miss out on the sense of what I am reading. This made it bad for me in school. When I could not understand, sometimes I would try harder but I got discouraged when it had no effect, so I would just mess about.

Reading out in class, or aloud to anyone is the worst, because I often miss out letters, and pronounce things wrong, like if I am reading three I might say tree instead, which really annoys me, as I know I have said it wrong because of the context.

My Dad and I have done some experimenting with colours on the computer, and two things to make the text readable really stand out.

The first, which is how I have written my book, is to leave a space between each paragraph, which splits up a page into sections. Otherwise the page just looks like a white glaring sheet with black lines going across. The other thing is if we change the background to dark grey on the computer, and the lettering to white, it makes the words stand out. The letters seem to have more shape, and there is spacing between the words. Normally they look joined up to me, which is why I have so much trouble reading. My Dad's computer's word-processing program has yellow typing on a blue background, which is by far the easiest to read. My Smith Corona is white on blue, which is quite good too. This is one of the secrets why I am able to do so well on a word processor.

I am now going to try and describe what it feels like to be dyslexic.

Having dyslexia is like having a nerve that has gone wrong and I just can't make it go away. As I am writing this it is hard for me, because I think it is impossible to describe your feelings in full. The whole idea of feelings is that while you can feel them, you can't make people feel them by using words, they must feel them too. So I think the secret of dyslexia is only inside the people who have it. Normal people cannot understand at all, so it is really hard for them to help dyslexic people overcome the problem.

In primary school I used to sit alongside a computer that was never used, and I would try my best because I really thought I was stupid. I just felt I wasn't good enough – I was no good at reading, writing, art or other things like that. I felt very left out but I made up for it in sport, because I was good at sport and everyone would pick me for their team, which made me feel much better.

When I first had my word processor at school I used to hate it, because it was quite big and heavy, as it was a portable word-processing typewriter with its own built-in printer. I had to carry it around and everyone would see and ask me what it was, so sometimes I would 'forget' to get it from the office. Then – luckily, I guess, for me – the only powerpoint packed up in one of the classrooms where I used my PWP a lot, and it took five months for the school to fix it. So we changed the word processor for the new portable model which had just come out. It is much smaller and fits in my bag. This makes it much easier, and now I take it to all my lessons.

At first I was very nervous about what everyone would say about my having a PWP. Some people hated me because I had it, but I had to cope with that and now everyone in my class accepts it as being normal.

My Dad, who is busy writing his part of the book, has just asked me if I can tell the time on a normal clock. This made me realise that I can't, and it is one of the things that has made me feel stupid, though I have never told my Mum or Dad. It has never been a problem because I have always been able to read a digital clock.

I have just had a break, and I asked my Mum to teach me how to tell the time. It's really quite easy, you just have to say the right hand side is past, and the left hand side is to, so if the little hand is on the six and the big hand is on the four, it's twenty past six.

Dyslexia is like being really stupid, which you're not, and frustrated all the time, because you can't write what you want to say in a way that other people can understand. The problem for me is that my hand will not do what my brain is telling it to, no matter how hard I try. It is like trying to write blindfolded with handcuffs on and having to look most of the words up in a normal dictionary, and then still spelling them wrong. Writing takes all my concentration, especially if I want to write neatly – if I let it flow out, like it does on the PWP, you can't read it.

With my PWP, I don't have that problem and my hands fly over the keys – typing just comes naturally to me now, like writing does for other people, and with the automatic dictionary I know I will spell the words right. The one problem it doesn't help me with is confusing words that sound alike: I often put write instead of right or now instead of know.

It would be agony for you if you suddenly got dyslexia. To you it would be like reading and writing in a foreign language.

For me knowing that I am not normal, and not being able to do the things that other people take for granted, is what I hate most and what really gets me down. The worst time for me is when I think I will get nowhere in life, and that because of my problem, I will end up on the street. I think the most important thing in life is to have a roof over your head, and not go hungry.

I feel sad to know that I will never overcome dyslexia fully. What I am thankful for is that the technology is available that has changed my life forever. However, I will always feel sad inside and know that no-one can stop that, not even the best teacher in the world. So if you have dyslexia just keep trying to conquer it. Think of all the things you are good at, not things you are bad at. Don't give up, because dyslexia is not the main problem, it is the feeling of frustration that you really have to overcome!

PARIS'S
SHORT STORIES

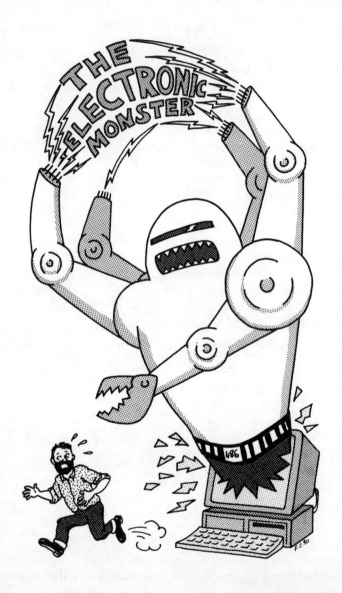

THE ELECTRONIC MONSTER

CHAPTER 1
ADDICTION

The year is 1990 and computers rule the world. Everyone has one. I am even writing this story on one, which is about my Dad who became addicted to his computer. It all started when my parents found out I was dyslexic, which is when my Dad became interested in computers.

Because I am dyslexic, he bought me a computer so that I could read what I was writing, because my handwriting is so bad. When he got the computer I changed completely, because I could read what I had written. My Dad then also decided to buy a computer so he could draw his designs much easier, and it worked. But! it was *bad*, because he became addicted to it and couldn't stop working on it. He would work until he fell asleep at night.

His family would keep telling him to stop, but he refused to listen to them, until it got so bad, that he stopped work and he just sat at his computer all day. He didn't even draw new ideas. He would just fiddle and print bits of nothing. Then his family started to put together the bits of the drawing. It made a picture of a huge electronic monster, and when his family looked at the monster, it winked at them.

One day my Dad saw a laser light coming from the printer, which was flashing. As he looked at it, he heard a sucking noise, then, suddenly, he was lifted from his chair and sucked into the printer.

When he arrived it was dark at first, then as his eyes grew accustomed to the light, he could see lights and wires all around him. He walked along a narrow path and as he came to the end of it, there was a slope. He decided to slide down and see what was at the bottom.

He started sliding down, and it got steeper and steeper until it seemed that it was going to go almost vertical. So, as he was passing many ledges, he reached out and grabbed one and scrambled on to it.

At the other end of the ledge there was a small door, so he opened it and crept inside. He walked along a dark passage which led to a great big room, at the other end of which was a hole in the ground. He slid himself through the hole and came out into a gigantic room. In the room there was nothing but a ladder, so he climbed up it, and found himself in a place with great big rollers, which he guessed was the paper feed-out when you finished printing.

He could see through the rollers and saw his son writing something on the computer. As he watched, a piece of paper was coming up behind him, and it looked like it was going to push him into the rollers, but he bent down to pick up his watch he had dropped, and it just missed him.

After he had watched his son for a bit, he carried on walking until he came to a great big rope which he guessed was the power lead. He waited until the power was switched off and then he slid down the wire. At the bottom, he found he had arrived at the monitor.

He was now at the top of the monitor, so he had to get down to the bottom, to the computer, so he could escape out of the disc drive. By doing this he thought he would return to normal size. He could be wrong, but he thought he would try as hard as he could to get out of there, if he couldn't he would destroy it so it couldn't poison his son's mind like it had his.

CHAPTER 2
THE LAND

At the top of the monitor he could see down for miles and the only way down was to climb down the circuit board. The circuit board went to the bottom of the monitor. So he started to climb down the circuit board until he reached a ledge where he settled down to sleep.

After he had been sleeping for an hour or so, he woke up to find a midget curled up in his arms, sleeping. He pushed the midget off, and the little midget woke with a start. My Dad said, 'Who are you and what is your name?'

The midget replied, 'My name is Chip and I live in this computer. Some people say I make it work, but all I do is sit here and sleep.'

Chip had a rectangular body, with a smooth back, but with loads of pins sticking out of his front. He had a little round head, short arms and legs, with no hands or feet. Although he had a hard shell-like back, his front was very soft and tender. He neither likes, nor is very good at fighting, but he is a very fast runner. If he hit you at speed, however, no matter how big you are he would knock you over.

My Dad started to ask questions about what it was like being a chip, but Chip said he didn't feel like answering any personal questions. So instead Dad asked if he knew the way to the disc drive, and Chip said he did, but it was dangerous and they would be in great danger if they went. My Dad said that he must go because his family's life was at stake. So they set off and they soon reached the bottom, where there was a wire. Chip jumped down and my Dad followed him.

They both landed at the end of the wire and the chip told him that they were in the main computer case. My Dad looked around and saw all the different bits of the machine that he had seen when he was big. Chip took him along a long narrow tunnel which led them into a room full of mirrors and there, in one of the mirrors, was the electronic monster.

The monster looked huge and very scary. It had five arms, one with pincers that it used to pick up things, the other four with spikes that it used to stab things with. Its round head had no neck, but moulded into its body, and it had a red glowing line for its eye. It had four legs with spikes at the end to support its short body. Its wings were of woven wire, and its teeth when the slit opened were razor sharp. It had on a belt made from microchips, with a large one for the buckle. The surface of its body looked alive, with flashing lights and buttons all over it.

The two of them stood still. They blinked and as they looked around they saw nothing, as the monster had disappeared.

Chip said, 'At the end of this room, there is a door, and once we are through it you can get out through the disc drive. Then you can help your family escape from the curse.' As they started to walk towards the door, the monster jumped out on to my Dad and tried to scratch his eyes out. Chip, however, ran at the monster and knocked it over.

They ran for the door, but somehow the monster had beaten them to it, and was blocking their path. They split up and the monster started to chase my Dad. He ran and ran, and then suddenly he stopped. He turned around and stuck out his leg, and the monster tripped and skidded along the floor, hitting some mirrors. They shattered and the monster was cut by the glass, so Chip and my Dad ran out the door, into the disc drive.

At the mouth of the disc drive the two friends shook hands, but as my father was going to jump the monster appeared, and it leapt at my Dad. But Chip pushed my father out of the mouth of the disc drive and got in the monster's way. As he fell my Dad could hear the screams coming from inside the computer.

As my Dad hit the floor, he started to grow. When he was half grown, he picked up the nearest object to him and smashed the computer to bits. As he turned away the monster escaped through a mousehole in the wall and went on to the next computer.

The moral of the story is always keep your disc drives shut, as this is how the monster gets in!

SURVIVAL

'Could you please fasten your seat belts?' the loudspeaker said.

My mother, little sister and I all did up our seat belts. The plane took off but after about fifteen minutes the plane started to run into a bit of trouble. We held tight to each other and saw that we were going to crash.

People were crying and screaming. The captain came out and said, 'Could you all sit down?'

Then there was a 'bang'. We must have hit something, and I saw the captain fly back.

I woke only to find my mother lying dead on top of me. I pushed her off and turned to my sister. She was crying. I comforted her and then I saw that everyone was dead. I later realised that my mother had saved us by lying over me and my sister.

We got out of the plane and sat down. I said to my sister, 'We better go to the village.' We walked down to a small village and asked for food and water, but when I said we were American they threw us out. They said we were dangerous and no one would help us.

We found a shelter and went to sleep. In the middle of the night I was awakened by a noise. I picked up a stick and said, 'Come out, wherever you are.'

After a while a small Japanese boy came out and said, 'I can help. I can take you to an American camp.' He had a bag of food with him, so as we were starving we all tucked in, and then settled down to sleep for the rest of the night.

The next day we set out for the American camp which was many miles away. That day we walked for twelve hours, hiding whenever a patrol came by. By that time it was getting dark so the Japanese boy, whose name was Foo, said, 'We will sleep here for the night.' Next morning we awoke to find Foo cooking some fish. After the breakfast of fried herrings, we set out again.

Coming to a road block Foo decided we should go around it, so we headed up a slope to a large tree. As we did so, a Japanese soldier spotted Foo and opened fire. We could not afford to lose Foo so I sneaked up behind and hit the soldier over the head with a large stick. Foo then grabbed the gun and shot him. Dropping the gun, we all ran through the trees until we had passed the road block. After we were a safe distance away we found a stream, where Foo caught some more fish, which we cooked and ate, and then we went to sleep.

In the middle of the night we were captured by Japanese soldiers and taken off to their camp, and thrown into a damp room with no lights.

Next morning I found myself in a wooden hut by myself. Then the door opened and my sister was thrown in. She was crying and said they had been beating her and she couldn't understand her captors because they were speaking in Japanese. I said, 'That Japanese scum, I just knew Foo was a spy,' but secretly I didn't believe it and I still trusted him.

Suddenly two guards came in and said, in English, 'Come with us. Our leader wants to see you.' They picked us up and took us to the biggest hut, and threw us on the floor. When we looked up we got the shock of our lives, there was our father. He said, 'Come children, come and say hello to your Dad.' My little sister stood up, and just as she started to run towards him, I stopped her and said, 'Don't you see, he is on the enemies' side?'

My father looked at me with pure hate in his eyes, and said to the guards, 'Take him back to the hut.'

My sister said, 'No! Don't! If you take him you take me too.'

'Very well,' said my father, and the guards took us both back to the dark hut.

Next day my father came into the hut where we were being held, and said that he had meant to kill my mother. 'All the seat belts were tampered with except yours, so that you would be the only ones not killed. Instead of thanking me for saving you, you have decided to hate me, so I will just have to kill you.'

He then called the guards and they took us out to a firing squad. Just as we were about to be shot, a big explosion shook the camp. In the smoke and the confusion came Foo, who ran and cut our ropes, and set us free. We ran off into the forest, but it did not take them long to realise that we had escaped and my father sent guards after us, but we managed to hide in some trees and they went off in the opposite direction.

The next day, many miles away, we made a camp so we had somewhere we could sleep and eat.

The next day we started our plan of revenge against our father. We stole guns from the soldiers in the camp, and soon had enough guns and other weapons to fight our father. The next night we set up outside his base, with forty guns, all set to go off when we pulled a piece of string, so that they couldn't shoot us. We left my sister there and Foo and I went out with bazookas and machine guns to start the fight. After surprising them and using all our shells, we ran back to my sister, where we set all the guns off. We knew we couldn't win as there were too many of them, so we ran off into the forest, where we lived until the war was over.

WIZARD GIRL

There was a flash of light, the white knights galloped across the drawbridge and into the forest. The knights had been told by the king of Aron to destroy the wizard of Galan so he could rule the land.

The wizard had been warned by his spies in the king's palace, and was preparing his magic to stop the white knights. White knights, however, could not be stopped by ordinary magic, they had to be stopped with great spells. The white knights had been created by magic, by the evil king of Aron. They had magical powers themselves and could only be destroyed by the black knights. The black knights had been created by the wizard to guard the land of Galan against the evil white knights.

Unfortunately, the wizard could not kill the white knights, he could only stop their advance temporarily. The trouble was that the black knights were on a crusade in the south fighting the Quillians, while the wizard lived in Rasco Castle in the east.

As the white-armoured knights galloped into the castle, the wizard created an illusion of a dragon so big the white knights turned and rode for their lives.

The wizard sent a message to the black knights telling them to return, because the king of Aron had sent the white knights to kill him. As the messenger left, the white knights returned and struck the wizard to the floor, but they left before he was dead and he managed to release his magical powers into a little girl who was passing the courtyard where the wizard had been stuck down.

The girl, who was an orphan, stood crying in the middle of the courtyard next to where the wizard lay dead.

Soon the black knights returned, and found the girl, whose name was Arrett, wrapped in the wizard's clothes, but the wizard had disappeared. The black knights realised that the girl had received the magic and that soon, although she did not realise it, she would be the most powerful woman in the world.

As Arrett grew up, she became more and more powerful, until at sixteen she decided on a quest to avenge the death of the wizard.

She rode with her black knights out of her castle to the king of Aron's castle. When they arrived the black knights flew up the walls of the castle with the aid of their golden wings, which sprouted from their feet. At the top they bombarded the castle defenders with their magical fire-balls which instantly vaporised the king of Aron's army. They then flew down into the courtyard where they fought off the rest of the guards who were defending the keep.

They made their way up a winding staircase until at the top they came to a door. They burst in and there was the king surrounded by the white knights. The black knights charged the white knights with their swords, because as both had been created by magic, it meant that their magic could only be used on mortal people, not on each other. The wizard girl walked through the men who were fighting and up to the king and said, 'You killed the wizard and now it is my destiny to kill you!' She then used her magic to lift up the king and throw him out of the window and down into the moat, to be eaten by his own pet crocodiles.

THE GREAT STORM

In 1990, there was a storm to end all storms. It was made by a professor who could make the weather change at any time. One day he thought of an idea to stop all weather so that he could make each season perfect, for crops to grow so there would be no famine.

He thought that if he directed the weather towards the centre of the earth, it would make the world spin around until all the weather for the next ten years had been lost into time. The idea was to insert the professor's perfect weather into time, and after the ten years had passed the weather would revert to normal. So the professor started to work out how he would catch the storm and direct it towards the centre of the earth.

First of all he programmed his computer to fire his special Z-rays, to catch a storm and direct it at the centre of the earth. He then went about his business and waited until the next storm. He was in a supermarket doing his shopping, when he heard on a radio that there was a storm coming to Miami.

So the professor ran out of the store, got into his car and drove to his house at high speed, to where he kept his computer. He typed in code 749-129-367 and the machine started to hum. After a few minutes the house began to shake and then spin. The professor ran outside, fell and knocked himself out.

When he awoke he was surrounded by people asking him what had happened. He looked around and saw that everything was OK. So he got up and went inside his house only to find that it was not his, but an old woman's, who he had bought it from four years previously. He then decided to go to his old house where he could get the bits to make a machine which would crystal-leap him back to 1990 so he could alter his weather machine.

21

So he set off for his old house where he used to live. When he arrived he saw himself get into a cab and drive off. So he ran up to his old apartment, got the spare key from a neighbour and went into his old house. In the house there was a lab with all the things he needed to get back home.

He raced around getting all the bits together and after about three hours he had finished. Just as he finished he saw himself coming through the door, so he hid behind a door, and when he saw himself going into the kitchen, he jumped out from his hiding place and pushed the button to take him back to his own time.

He arrived back in 1990 in a flash of blinding light. He then rushed into his house and stopped the machine and suddenly, everything was back to normal again.

The moral of this story is 'Don't mess with Mother Nature'.

BABY-SNATCHERS

One of the biggest newspaper stories of 1990 was the case of the baby-snatchers. It all started one morning in London, with a woman who was shopping in Tesco's with her baby. She had left the baby in a pram while she had gone off to the bread counter. When she returned all she saw was a hooded person running off into the distance.

A few days after the snatching, at Scotland Yard they received a phone call, saying that the baby was safe but he would kill the baby if the ransom wasn't paid. The chief of Scotland Yard told his men to search for a baby anywhere and the mother not to tell the press.

So life went on and more and more babies went missing. Soon over twenty babies were missing and over £5,000,000 was being demanded in ransom.

The chief of Scotland Yard was pulling his hair out over the baby-snatcher, so he told the press and put up wanted notices everywhere for the return of the babies. The reward money for each baby was £5000 pounds. This was so the man who stole the babies could hand them in and get the reward.

After two weeks they had still not heard from the baby-snatcher, so they thought the babies were dead. However, they weren't, as they had been taken to a big house and were being looked after like kings. The baby-snatcher had no intention of killing them. He thought that if he kidnapped them the parents would look after them better.

So one dark night he went out and put all the babies back in their rightful homes, where they were looked after better than ever.

So this story is to all you uncaring parents, that if you don't want your baby taken from you, take good care of it or the 'baby-snatcher' might pay *you* a visit.

HEAVEN

The waves crashed down on the front of the three-mast ship, the *Bloody Mary*. Men were being thrown over the side screaming as they plunged into the darkness of the black sea.

In the mist the crew could see the outline of a Russian ship. It fired its cannons at them, but missed. The *Bloody Mary* was an English ship which had been thrown off course and was now heading for Russia.

The two ships fought bravely, but the English ship went down. The ten crew members who were left escaped in a long boat and were now heading for Turkey.

The crew who escaped were the captain, a Professor Sharr and eight sailors. When they arrived in Turkey, a French ship was waiting for them, and as soon as they landed they were taken prisoner and put on a ship for France.

Before they arrived, however, an English stowaway set them free and they escaped into the night. After ten hours swimming, they spied an island which they headed for. On the island, they found food and shelter. Every day they would go out hunting for food. On one of these hunts a sailor found a hole, and next to it there was an inscription, so he went to get the others.

When they arrived at the hole, Professor Sharr read the inscription and it said, 'Whoever manages to survive the long descent and the maze at the bottom will end up in Heaven.'

So everyone gathered all the food and water they could find and started on the long journey to the place where no man or woman had ever been and lived to tell the tale.

As the first sailor entered the darkness, he could feel a slimy liquid on the walls, and as he went lower it got slimier and slimier until it got so slimy he could barely hold on. However, he managed to hold on and eventually the slime went away. The others joined him and they carried on down.

As they went deeper, it got darker and darker and the fire torches went out, so they just had to feel their way. Every so often they would stop for a drink or food. They had been descending for several hours when they came to a tunnel. A voice was coming from inside and it said, 'This way to Heaven!' They could see a bright light at the end, so the first sailor stepped into the tunnel and a door closed behind him. They heard screams and then the door opened again and he was gone.

As they went deeper and deeper, they kept on coming to different tunnels with different voices all welcoming them to heaven. One by one the sailors went in, and were gone just like the one before. When they had passed all the tunnels, only the captain, Professor Sharr and three sailors were left. They continued on down, until they came to a platform with a long tunnel. Here they rested on the platform for a long time, before they started down the tunnel.

The tunnel had holes in the floor and ceiling. As the men walked down it, spikes started to come out of the ceiling and floor. Just as the last man was about to get out of the tunnel, a door closed and he was spiked.

They all turned from the tunnel and looked at the giant maze which lay ahead of them. In the middle of the maze was a white glow, which they guessed was Heaven. They started down the hill towards the maze, when they were stopped by a red baby dragon and it said, 'I can get you through the maze if you get me the ice crystal.' The dragon took them to the cave which had the ice crystal in it. What they did not know, was that it was more dangerous getting the ice crystal out of the cave than going through the maze.

As they entered the cave, a door closed the entrance to the cave. As they walked along they saw scratch marks on the wall made by a giant creature. Suddenly they heard a roar and a giant beast appeared. It had an ape's head, giraffe's neck, human body, hawk's wings and Tyrannosaurus Rex's legs.

This beast was really ugly and it said, 'Yes? Can I help you?'

The men stared at the beast and said, 'Yes! We would like the ice crystal.'

The dragon roared and said, 'Everyone comes here for that.' The beast then tried to kill the men, but they managed to fight it off while one of them grabbed the ice crystal. They made for the door, and the beast seeing them threw a cannon ball at them, but it missed and hit the door, breaking it down and they managed to escape outside.

They gave the dragon the crystal and it took them by using its special magic through the maze to the centre where they met God.

Suddenly they all realised that everyone in Heaven wasn't eating and drinking and having a good time, they were all working. They said to God, 'Why are they working?'

God replied, 'They did not work on Earth, so they are making up for their laziness now.'

To all you people out there, remember, Heaven just might have a few surprises in store for you!

TRY THE TRI STAR

Georgie and Freddie ran to the gates of the fun fair, but the man stopped them at the gate and asked them for their money. They didn't have any, so they ran round the back and crept in through a hole, which they had done since they were four years old. This is because they had never had enough money to buy a ticket, but they knew that once they were in, all the rides were free.

As they squeezed through the fence, they saw a sign saying 'Try the Tri Star'. It pointed to the right, so the boys followed the arrow and soon came to a spinning ride which spun round and round and then, still spinning, went through a dark tunnel, and then corkscrewed back over the top of the tunnel again to the start.

The two boys ran up and grabbed their seats. The ride started! As it went round and round, the boys found themselves coming out of their seats and suddenly there was a flash of blinding light and they looked around and saw they were not on the ride, but in a desert.

As they looked across the desert, they heard a noise behind them. Turning around they saw small men made out of sand, wearing silver body armour. The men had a type of laser whip which they used for striking people. Georgie and Freddie were taken away down into a tunnel which went deep into a sand dune. Inside they came to an enormous room where a giant sand beetle towered over them.

The giant beetle said to the two boys, 'You are spies who have come from our enemies who live on the Forest Moon, and you have been sent here to find out what our "secret weapon" is!'

'No! that is not true, we are from Earth and we were brought here by mistake and we can't get back,' said Georgie.

'Why do you lie, take them away,' said the giant beetle, who had a shiny black shell with giant pincers on the side of its head and suckers on its legs.

The guards took the two boys to a cave, deep at the bottom of the underground city, locking them up with a 'man' with four arms. He said to them, 'I can help you, as I have built a secret passage out of here. I can take you to safety and help you get home.' The three companions set off down the narrow tunnel, which eventually came out on the surface. They ran off into the dark night. Soon they reached the man's hide-out and they all sat down for something to eat. They ate a mushy mixture which tasted like the smell of new shoes.

After dinner, they talked about all the things that were going on in Zem, the land which Georgie and Freddie had mysteriously arrived in. They talked for Zeckies (Zem time: One Zeckie = 1.5 Earth hours) before going to bed. Next morning they were woken up early by Mit, their dinner companion, and taken to where they could see the sandmen rounding up the Milids (the four-armed people) in a little village, and putting them into cages. Freddie said, 'Where are they taking them?'

'They will be used as slaves in the crystal mines,' said Mit. 'The crystal is for making a weapon so powerful that the sandmen can conquer other worlds like Earth.'

The two boys then decided to help the four-armed people and stop the sand people. Mit took them to a place where they could get weapons to fight the sand people, and they set off for the mines. Reaching the mines, they dealt with a patrol of two sandmen. Georgie and Freddie put on their armour, so they would not be recognised, and set off for the entrance to the mine.

On arriving at the entrance, they walked in, and inside they saw the Milids being whipped and beaten. Georgie and Freddie could not stand it, so they secretly started to release the Milids. Then they stormed the men inside the mine, killing them. They then took their weapons, went outside and killed all the sand people.

Then they made their way to the crystal tower where the weapon was being built. They waited for their chance to get inside the tower. This came when the guards fell asleep, so they seized their chance, killed them and made their way to the weapon. They fought and killed some guards, and then placed laser bombs on the weapon, and blew it up, when they got clear of the mine.

Outside, a battle was going on between the Milids and the sandmen. However, the Milids soon won, and there was much celebrating. The two boys wanted to go home, so Mid took them back to the place where they had arrived. They found themselves back on the ride again. When it finished they got off, and ran back home.

The next year they came back, but the 'Tri Star' had gone.

THATCHER'S ASSASSINATION

It is the first of January, 1991 – the year of Thatcher's murder.

The people plotting against her were the joint Labour and IRA group. As they put their plan to kill Thatcher into action, the first thing they did was gas the policeman outside. Then they tied him up.

The IRA kicked down the door and ran in, firing their machine guns. They ran up the stairs past all the dead bodies which had already been killed by fire from their Labour partners.

Then, out of nowhere came SAS men firing their machine guns. The few of the IRA who were still left carried on towards the PM's room. As they neared the PM's door, her secretary pulled a pistol out of a drawer, but was killed before he could use it.

Thatcher ran to a corner and said, 'Please don't kill me! Please don't kill me!'

The IRA man said, 'Shut up, and sit down.'

The Prime Minister sat down, and said, 'Do you want money?'

'No, we want you dead.'

Then the man brought up a gun to her face and pulled the trigger.

Out popped a sign saying 'BANG'.

Then he said, 'Smile, you're on Candid Camera.'

1989

This is the year of disaster in the economic world. I am a small business man, just a small fish in a big pool. But there were others who went right under.

First there was Jeff who was rich and a happy family man when the crash came. It turned him into a bundle of nerves. His marriage broke up and he is now a street cleaner, because what little money he had left he lost to his ex-wife.

Then there's Gerald. He lost his house, his car and his business. Now he lives in a council flat in the East End, working part-time as a cleaner in a pub.

Here comes the one I feel most sorry for. He had an argument with his boss when the crisis was at its peak and was sued for everything he had. Now he sleeps rough in Leeds, with nothing but the shirt on his back.

But when the biggest company in the world went bankrupt, no less than fifty million people were out of work. But the one who came off worst was the owner, because he had no skills other than running that business. So after he was turned out without one penny to his name, he wandered the streets. And when night came he stood outside Putney train station asking for a penny so he could buy a crust of bread.

THE GREAT CHASE

The sound of sirens could be heard. The two robbers ran out of the bank and into their car, a blue Ford. The cops turned the corner and started after them.

The Ford came out into the main road, skidded and made several cars spin out of control. One car went flying into a manure lorry and manure went on several people.

The police came round the corner, and sped off after the Ford on to the motorway. As the Ford came towards exit fourteen, two more patrol cars started after the Ford. An hour later, there were eleven patrol cars and two motorbikes after the robbers.

Then the Ford turned on to the other lane and went up the wrong way. Cars started skidding and rolling over. Then the two motorbikes came alongside the Ford. The Ford swerved, knocking off first one, then the other. One of the motorbikes went straight into a caravan, and they both blew up.

The Ford decided to go off the road. It bumped up and down, until it came to a river. The only way across was to jump off a small loading bay. The robbers stepped on the gas and managed to make it to the other side. However the leading police car stopped on the docking bay, but the car behind did not, and neither did the rest. They were all in the river.

The Ford stopped at a gas station, and the robbers stole a red Rover. The police got the message that they had switched cars, and a road block was set up. As they neared it, the robbers speeded up, and went straight through it. But the police turned and fired. The two robbers were killed instantly. Their car went into a tree and it blew up. Then the big clear up began.

THE ANIMALS' REVOLT

It all started in a zoo. The cleaner there was an animal hater and whenever he went into the monkeys' cage, he poked and hit them.

One day, the cleaner came as usual but when he went into the monkeys' cage, out came all the monkeys, hitting the man. Then they escaped and the man ran off out of the zoo.

The monkeys went around the zoo setting free all the animals.

As the first of them came out on to the street, people screamed and ran off down the road. The animals ran into the road, hitting cars, climbing lamp-posts and pushing down rubbish bins.

But no tarantulas got loose.

The animals stampeded across the land, setting free more and more animals until they took over the whole country.

Only one place was left untouched by the animals and that was a small island off the coast of France.

Because all the people on that island were kind to animals, the animals made them their royal family and they lived in harmony.

But everywhere else the animals used people for their food and kept some as pets.

JOURNEY TO THE CENTRE OF THE EARTH

The journey started when Doctor Duncan called a few of us to the convention. He told us that we should meet in a bar in London. When everyone had arrived, the doctor said that he was planning a journey – a journey to the centre of the earth. Anyone who wanted to come should stay but those who didn't should leave now. Quite a lot of men stood up and went.

The people who were left were Professor Plum, Arnold White, Jenny Summers, oh! and me, Paris Innes.

The doctor said that we should travel light and that we would leave for India on 20th June. June came and soon it was the day for us to board the plane, which was at 9 am.

We arrived in India at 4pm. The next day we started digging with the machine the doctor had invented and we soon came to some caves.

It was getting hot as we went through lots of passages. But by this time, the heat was not the only difficulty we faced. One of the men who had been at the meeting in London, had got together his own band of cut-throats and bandits and they were now following us.

As the doctor's party rounded a corner we saw a river of lava, crossed by an almost ruined stone bridge. Professor Plum stepped on it first and it fell, taking him into the lava.

Jenny Summers had fallen and was hanging on to a rock. Arnold and I helped her up.

We all decided that we should camp round the corner and we settled down to sleep. But the bandits had caught up. As we slept, they crept up, took us prisoner and tied us up. The leader and most of his gang continued on. They made a rope bridge and got across.

Two men were left to guard us but after about half an hour, I tripped one of them up and Arnold tripped the other. We got free, knocked them out and ran over the rope bridge, taking their guns with us.

We managed to catch up with the others and were just about to shoot them when Arnold slipped and they saw us. They opened fire but we returned it and hit one of them. They ran off in the opposite direction, so we cautiously started after them.

'Bang!' Arnold was shot in the arm. But we fired back and killed both of them. We ran on until we caught up with the first of the last group. Jenny fired at the man. We saw him fall and we left him there as we ran on.

It was getting hotter by the minute, until we saw a huge fire in front of us. Then we ran and ran faster and faster until we heard screams.

We stepped back and we saw the bandits covered in fire. We saw a hole in the roof and there was the bandit leader. We climbed up to him, until there we were, at the centre of the earth.

IDEAL SCHOOL

My ideal school would have lifts worked by robots and everybody would work with computers.

The entrance would be electronic and each member of the school would carry an electronic card which would be read by the entrance computer as you came in, so there would be no need for a register.

The building would be white and all the edges would be rounded off.

The teachers would be robots and the dinners would be self-service.

All the cleaning would be done by robots and if you dropped litter the robots would make you pick it up.

If the robots were vandalised they would take video pictures of their attacker, so that the person would be found and made to pay.

The grounds of the school would all be greenery and trees.

The word processors would be Smith Corona. Everyone would have a name tag.

If there was a fire, it would be quickly detected by sensors which would call the fire brigade and close fire-doors automatically. Robots would search the building and take a computer record of who was there.

For sport you would get changed and go through register doors and a robot would take you outside for your sports lesson.

Everyone would carry around a pocket electronic timetable which would bleep when you went into the wrong class.

And that is my school for the future.

THE REAL DISCOVERY OF TUTANKHAMEN

The two boys and the girl stood outside of their hotel in Calmar, looking across the desert, when they heard a shout, 'Ben, Sean, Janet! Come and help your mother in the bedroom.'

The three children ran up the stairs to help their mother pack her trunk.

'Why do you have to go back to London?'

'Because of my job, darling.'

Later, the children's father told them to go out and play a game, so they went outside and along came a van. The people in the van were American and their names were Fred and Frank. They said they would take them to the swimming pool.

So the children got into the van and they were taken along a rough road. Fred had black hair, a sweaty, wrinkled face, and was very thin. He had a high, crackly voice. Frank was a large man and he had a scar over his left eyebrow.

They were turning the eighth bend when the men stopped the car and said, 'Get out now.'

'But we are in the middle of nowhere,' said Sean.

Frank pushed them out of the van and drove off. The children were left standing next to a pyramid, but as they did not know what a pyramid was, they went inside to see if anybody would help them.

As they went into the first passage it was dark and damp. They turned left, then right, then two more lefts until they came to a stairway. Ben went up the first step, the second, then the third but, as he stepped on the fourth, the staircase went flat and Ben slid down. Next time he ran and made it to the top, so did Janet and Sean.

At the top of the stairs, they found themselves in a room with treasures made of gold and silver. Sean, a 'Leo' with ginger hair, was the most nervous one. Ben was quite big and not so nervous. Janet was a skinny person with a mouth as big as a cheetah.

Sean leant against the wall and a door opened up, which they all went through except Sean, who said he would keep watch outside.

Janet and Ben were in a room with a stone coffin in the middle. Janet went up to the coffin and said, 'Give me a hand with the lid.'

Ben helped her lift the lid and inside they found a man all wrapped in bandages. Janet screamed – but not because of the body. It was a man who had grabbed her from behind. He took them outside and their father was there, waiting for them to take them home.

There you have it! The real discovery of Tutankamen.

CHRISTMAS

A long time ago in a land far away there lived a man and his children. The children's mother had died in an accident with a sleigh.

One bright Christmas morning, the children went out looking for a Christmas tree. They had been walking for about ten minutes when they came to a clearing with a tree in the middle. The little girl touched the tree and disappeared. The little boy jumped in alarm, but then he touched the tree and he disappeared too.

The boy found himself in the clouds. When he looked down he felt dizzy, so he stood up straight and started walking.

Quite soon he saw a small elf-like thing. As he approached, the elf spun round. 'What do you want?' it said.

'I want to know where I am,' the boy said.

'You are in Cloud City,' said the elf.

The boy looked round. 'I want to go back home,' he said. 'And I want to find my sister.'

'I know someone who knows,' said the elf.

'Take me to him,' the boy said.

The elf picked up a strange-looking bag and said, 'Follow me.'

The boy followed until the elf came to a strange door in the clouds and knocked. Out came a massive giant who bent down to speak to the boy.

'What do you want?' asked the giant.

The boy said, 'I want to find my sister.'

'Come in,' said the giant. He showed the boy and the elf into a long, grim tunnel. They walked until they came to a big door which the giant opened. As they went inside, the boy could hear music and then he saw a big party going on with Father Christmas right in the middle, smiling at his sister.

The children were put on a sleigh and were taken home, where they had a very merry Christmas.

LOST IN SPACE

The invading troops had landed and were making their way towards the base. It was Red Alert!

My name is Corporal Bates and I was getting the escape pod ready when a missile hit the side of the base. I was thrown into the pod and I hit the take-off button. The rockets fired and as I took off, I was knocked out. When I awoke I was lost in space.

A few days later I was nearly out of food when the computer detected an inhabited planet. I set course and as we approached I could see rivers and trees and the computer said, 'This is the planet Mender.'

My ship landed and the door opened. I came out with my gun because I didn't know what was on the planet. I walked towards the stream and tasted the water. It was good.

When I reached out to touch a fruit, a laser hit my hand. I turned and fired but missed and a voice said, 'Don't you take my crops.'

I said, 'Just one fruit?'

He said, 'Throw down your gun and walk out.'

I did as he said and saw that he was a green, slimy blob.

'Who are you?' it asked.

'I am Jeff,' I said.

The thing pushed me into his house.

'Please,' I said, 'give me food.'

The blob said to his wife, 'Fix him something.'

The blob's wife, as it were, busied itself making food. Then it put a bowl of green mush in front of me. I ate it and it tasted lovely. The blob then said, 'You must go.'

'But my ship has no fuel, please let me stay.'

'No,' the blob said.

'Oh, let him stay!' said its wife.

And the blob said, 'Yes.'

So I stayed there for twenty metrons. Then, one bright morning, there was a sound like thunder and a rocket appeared. I ran out and a door opened. Out came a rescue team to take me home.

I thanked the blobs and said 'goodbye' but, just before the ship took off, I jumped and I stayed with the blob family until I died.

THE GREAT BIKE RACE

It was Tuesday 4th February, 1486, the day of the Great Bike Race.

The competitors were Hareled Grimshor, the Lovelesses, Sir Morris the Sixth and Mr Albert Hemshor. They lined up for the start – Mr Grimshor on his smooth-running Z2, the Lovelesses on their 'Circle Cycle', Sir Morris on his own Morris Machine and Mr Hemshor with his Bicycle Combination.

When the gun went off and the bikes sped away, the first into the lead was Sir Morris. But they had not been going long when he slowed to take a corner and Mr Hemshor's Bicycle Combination took over as leader of the pack.

Soon they came to a pit stop. Sir Morris said to his mechanic, 'Get rid of Hemshor.'

They set off once again, and as Hemshor rounded the corner, he hit a giant rock and went flying into a bush. Then round came the others and they went slap bang into the stone – all except Sir Morris. After everyone had got back on their bikes, Hemshor was still in front but was followed closely by Sir Morris. When they came to their first hill Sir Morris had the advantage and, as they climbed it, he went out in front and Hemshor dropped right to the back.

In the last miles of the race, Sir Morris and Hemshor were still neck and neck when Sir Morris's men changed the signs. He came round a bend, took a short cut down a rough track and when he came out he was back in the lead.

Both men could see the finish line but Hemshor went faster and faster till he was neck and neck with Sir Morris.

When they both crossed the line, it was a photo finish. The two men lined up to hear the result and Mr Hemshor was declared the winner.

Mr Hemshor and his team jumped for joy. They drank champagne and they shook their opponents' hands. No one bothered to complain about Sir Morris's cheating because he lost anyway. Then the Hemshor team put their rosettes on their machine and rode the bike home in triumph.

THE BATTLE

This story takes place in a world like no other. My name is Gobe and I was searching for a new planet which is now called Earth. It was in the time zone when computers controlled the Earth and robots worked.

I was young and I was in a new ship in which I had been fighting the Gab and his evil force. One of their ships had damaged my engine and I was floating towards the earth. I could see satellites all round me and as I came into the Earth's atmosphere I saw nothing but trees and grass. I landed in what they call a cornfield. I was using my hover scoot to explore and that is when I met my friend, Mick.

He was riding a motorbike when he crashed into me, but we made friends and he took me to his house. I looked at his computer which was very primitive but then he showed me a skateboard and how to use it. I had a go and did a handplant off a half-pipe. Mick said I was 'rad'.

My landing had not been too good but I managed to contact home via the computer even though it was an early model. It needed so much power for the signals to reach home, that it interfered with the traffic lights and the electricity supply, and soon we had the FBI on to us.

We escaped on hover scoots but then I saw the Gab's ship land. They had sent mercenaries to kill me. I knew this because Mick killed one of them with a blow torch. We were on the run from the FBI, the Gab and Mick's mother. Mick was not so rad at scooting but we were able to move fast enough to keep ahead.

We made it back to my ship and Mick fought off the FBI and the

Gab while I fixed the engine. We lifted off into space and headed back home to my planet.

I can't wait to show them Mick and the skateboard.

A DAY IN THE LIFE OF A CAT

The day starts on the boy's bed. First, Charlie the cat gets up and has something to eat. He does a quick patrol of his territory which starts with his own garden. Then he goes over the wall to visit his neighbour who is called Peter. Together they check through his land first by just looking to see if anyone is there. Then they go round sniffing to double-check.

The two cats then split up and go hunting. Charlie finds a mouse. He crouches low, then pounces on his prey. He misses this time, but next time he may get lucky.

Charlie returns home for something to eat because he has not been successful with the mouse. He goes around the house looking for predators and is then about to have a sleep when he catches a glimpse of a cat in the garden.

He runs out to see who it is, but finds that it is only Peter. However, when they are out there they see a real enemy and go for the chase. Charlie is smacked in the paw, but not before inflicting a large scratch on the enemy cat, who runs away, hurt.

Peter gets Charlie home and Maggie (Charlie's master's Mum) takes him in the car to the vet who gives him some pills and orders him to rest. Charlie is not allowed out of the house for a whole week.

THE THREE WISHES

There once lived an orphan boy who had no relations whatsoever, so he just went around scrounging for his food.

One day he was looking for something to drink because he had just eaten some leftover chips with lots of salt on them. As he roamed the streets looking in dustbins, he came across a can – so he kicked it. The can span in the air and landed the right way up. But to Jimmy's astonishment, a cloud of smoke came out and out of the smoke emerged a man.

'Thank you,' said the man. 'I feel generous today so I will give you three wishes.'

The boy was so shocked he just stood and stared. 'I know this is Candid Camera,' he said.

But the man turned his head as if he was confused. 'Candid Camera? What is that?' he asked.

The boy took no notice and said, 'Do I really get three wishes?'

'What is your name?' asked the man, after a silence.

'Jimmy,' the boy said. There was a silence again while Jimmy wondered about this strange man. 'What is *your* name?' he asked.

'Oma,' said the man.

Then Jimmy shouted, 'I wish I had a car.'

Oma blinked twice and there was a car. Jimmy could hardly believe his eyes. He jumped into the driving seat to see if it was real, and Oma jumped in beside him. Jimmy was certain now that he was not dreaming. He drove away and the car felt real. Then he saw a police car behind them with a blue light flashing.

'I wish I had a driver,' said Jimmy – and there was a driver.

They pulled over because the police thought they had seen the boy driving.

'Sorry to have troubled you,' said the policeman, as he looked at the driver in amazement. Then, puzzled, he went back to his car.

'Now!' thought Jimmy. 'I know what I want! I want a thousand wishes!'

'You are being greedy,' said Oma 'and you lose all your wishes.'

Jimmy was sitting on the road with all the cars beeping at him. He walked off with nothing but what he started with – which was nothing.

THE HOUSE ON THE HILL

There was once a house on the hill in a place called Notting Hill. The whole area around the hill had been cleared for a giant new Tesco Superstore. However, just before this particular house was to be knocked down, it was inhabited by a squatter called Mr Plonker.

Here he was happy and he had many of his friends around, until after six months the Tesco man came around and said, 'You have to leave the house, Mr Plonker, because finally we have your eviction notice. We give you 48 hours to leave the hill.'

'I have no money to leave the hill,' said Mr Plonker.

'So get some,' said the Tesco man.

So Mr Plonker went out and, avoiding the Job Centre, he searched for a well paid job. After several hours he went to the Job Centre, even though it was a last resort.

When he got there, he looked for the most highly paid job which was a road sweeper.

'It comes with de luxe sweeping equipment and it is the best job we have,' said the girl at the desk in the Job Centre.

So, after the first two hours of sweeping, he asked his partner, who was a combination between a hippy, punk and a Brosette, 'How much do we get paid?'

'Well, man! We get about £100.' His partner laughed like a hippy and said, giving his best Bros imitation, 'Really! It's only nothing, nothing, nothing at all.'

'I can't get the money with this job, then,' said Plonker.

By now, however, it was too late. The deadline had been reached, so he went back to his house and packed up all his things and went back to the Sainsbury's office where he met his boss.

He said, 'You sure fooled those Tesco men, especially with your roadsweeping job. Here is what we agreed' (giving him a thick brown paper envelope), 'your new papers for your new identity, and the next assignment. Thanks to you we now have our new store open and nearly all Tesco's customers.'

THE DEATH OF SHERLOCK HOLMES

Holmes and I were on one of our most famous cases – The Stealing of the Crown Jewels. We were in Baker Street when I answered a ring at the door. It was a young lady who said her uncle was missing. I let her in to tell Holmes all about it and he said he would get on the case right away.

Now, Holmes is a tall, well brought up man with big bushy eyebrows and is not a man that turns down a challenge. I said to Holmes that we could not do two cases at once.

'My dear Watson, I fear that these two things are not just a coincidence.'

'What do you mean, Holmes?'

'I mean someone is trying to lead us away from our search for the Crown Jewels.'

The first thing we did was to visit the girl who had come to us. She lived as a tenant in an out-of-the-way back-street in East London. The door was opened to us by the landlord who was a fat, beer-bellied man with a fag in his mouth and stains on his vest. We walked up a shabby staircase and into her room. She was sitting on a chair in the corner. Her pretty face looked cold and even lifeless. Holmes went up to her and said, 'We would like to ask you some questions.'

There was a silence. I walked up to her and felt her pulse. I turned to Holmes and said, 'She's dead.'

'I'm going to call the police,' said Holmes. He went down the stairs and while he was away I examined the girl and found a dart in the dead girl's neck. When Holmes returned, I showed it to him.

'The Voodoo,' he mumbled.

'What?' I asked.

'Oh, nothing. Just a case I was on – one that was never solved.'

The next day, in Baker Street, a thirteen-year-old boy came to the house and said that his mother had gone missing.

'Stay here,' said Holmes to the boy. 'You might be in danger.'

We gave the boy a room. That night, Holmes went out and I was left to guard the boy. At about seven o'clock, the lights went out and the next thing I knew was that a sharp object hit me on the back of my head. I was knocked out.

Holmes woke me with whisky and said, 'Where is the boy?'

'Don't know,' I croaked. After I had told him what had happened, we went down to the police station and reported.

As we made our way home in the dark, and were turning into Baker Street, a bullet hit the pavement. Holmes and I started running. We got to our house and ran inside.

The next day Holmes came down the stairs and said to me, 'I think someone is trying to kill me.'

A few hours later, we went out to see whether the person who had shot at us had left any clues. As we got to the scene, Holmes saw a footprint. 'I now know who is trying to kill me,' he said.

'Who?' I said.

Then, suddenly, out came the little boy with a girl. He had the dart shooter and she had the gun. They both fired and Holmes was dead.

I turned and ran for my life. I reached the police station. I ran in and said, 'Come quickly! Holmes has been shot.' Three policemen ran with me back to where Holmes had been shot. But nothing was there. No blood, no body, no boy and no girl.

The police sergeant said, 'You will be getting a letter from the station, Mr Watson. About wasting police time.'

I was left there, feeling one minute as though I had imagined it all but another minute feeling as though it had all been real.

Later, I made my way back home and here I am writing the story, one year later . . . and still the mystery has not been solved.

HOW TO GET RID OF RUBBISH

The way to get rid of rubbish is to dig a hole and put the rubbish in. But the way I see it, we could get rid of it much more easily by using a new invention by a Doctor Labwith.

Now this invention takes rubbish and turns it into other goods like food, a TV or whatever you want. But for everything you take out, you must put something back in. No one knows why, but you do.

So Doctor Labwith sold one of the machines to a rich Arab. The doctor told the man that he must put something back in for everything he took out. The Arab said, 'Yes, yes,' and took the machine back to the Sudan.

But the Arab just did not put anything back into the machine. So after a year, the machine ate one of the Arab's wives. Then another. The Arab wondered about what the doctor had said to him.

One day the Arab came into the room where the machine was and saw that the machine had eaten all his wives. So the Arab ordered his servants to take the machine and burn it.

After three of his servants had been eaten they managed to burn the machine.

Meanwhile, Doctor Labwith had sold three more machines: one to an American film star, another to an English duke and a third to a Libyan terrorist.

The American film star put the machine in the back garden in a greenhouse. Well, the first thing that happened was that the pool was emptied and the gardener disappeared. Then the greenhouse went and then the film star himself was eaten.

The English duke lived in a big stately house with a cook, two chambermaids and his wife. Well, it started with the cook, then the chambermaids. Finally, he and his wife were eaten and I have been told that the machine ate the whole house inside out.

Then we come to the nastiest one of all – the terrorist. His family lived in a house on a hill in Libya. But the machine was in a warehouse just outside the city. First it ate the guards, then the warehouse and then it went up to where the terrorist lived and tried to eat them. But the family got away and I hear that they are being chased all over the world.

So if one of your friends goes missing, it might be that they have been eaten by the machine.

THE LOCH NESS MONSTER

To us the Loch Ness Monster is a fantasy, but it is not so to a small boy who lived on the side of Loch Ness. The little boy's name was Jamie McHagiss.

Early one morning he was walking along by the side of the loch, when a small ripple appeared on the surface. It got larger and then a huge shape emerged from the water.

It sent showers of water off its enormous lizard-like hide. As it came out of the water, towering over Jamie, it stared down at him.

Jamie squeaked, 'Please don't hurt me, Mr Monster.'

The monster said, 'Don't be afraid, I am not going to hurt you, as I want you to be my friend, as my friends are dying, and I want you to help me stop the people pumping all their sewage into the sea.'

Jamie said, 'What can *I* do to help?'

'Get all your friends to help you, and then go to the main sewage pump, and blow it up,' said the monster.

Jamie ran to get Jimmy and Robert, and then they all rounded up the other members of the gang. Eight in all. Each was given a list of things to get, like equipment such as rope, airguns and knives, money, and explosives.

When everyone was ready they waited until one o'clock in the morning, when they crept out of their houses and made their way to the airport.

Jamie borrowed his Dad's private plane (he had learnt to fly on his computer simulator) and they all flew to the private runway at Heathrow, where they hopped into his Dad's limo, and drove to the main sewage pump.

The first obstacle was the electric fence. They nailed a rope ladder to the floor and they threw it over the fence. They climbed up and jumped from the top and were then surrounded by dogs. These were, however, content with the lamb chops that were thrown to them, so they didn't attack.

The gang ran on until they reached the guard house, where they made the guards stand against the wall. Jimmy stood guard with his airgun while the others ran on to the pump.

When they arrived more guards appeared, shooting at them from behind, so the rest of the gang held them off while Jamie ran with the explosives towards the pump.

Just as he reached his goal, he was shot, and both the pump and Jamie went up in a ball of flames.

SUPER-BIKE 2000

This is the year of a radical new Super-bike. It is able to withstand rough treatment, has a streamlined front, with twenty speeds available.

It has a lie-back seat and no wheels, only air jets, which make it hover until you move them to a different angle which pushes the bike forward. It has extra boosters for getting up steep cliffs.

The lock works by recognising your palm print. If someone tries to steal it, the controls of the bike lock up and it also photographs the thief.

Steering is controlled by a joystick, and it has a maximum speed of 50 miles per hour. The speed of the Super-bike varies automatically, depending on the age of the driver, because the lock also recognises the age of the palm print.

They can be made into cars by linking them together, but as bikes they make travelling to work much easier, and would save people from being late for work.

It would change the entire transport and travel industry. People could also park without getting clamped, or getting a ticket.

Other versions could be made to be fold up, and another with fold-out wheels for the 'L' drivers. At night it has a button which you push which automatically covers it up.

THE BIRTH OF CHRIST

December 25th, 1989

In a small village in Ethiopia lived a man and his wife to be. One night the man, whose name was Joseph, was woken by an angel.

The angel said, 'Your wife Mary is going to have a child, a baby boy. Do not tell anyone! It is God's child, he will be the Son of God.'

So in time they got married, and when the baby was due they went to an air-raid shelter, as Ethiopia was at war. At midnight they went to the back of the shelter where there was a Texaco garage, and soon after their baby boy was born, who they named Jesus. The garage owner kindly gave them ten free coupons.

That night astrologers followed Rupert Murdoch's new TV satellite which stopped over the garage, which by now was surrounded by lots of unemployed newsmen writing reports.

The three astrologers who came brought gifts of guns, bullets and grenades.

The baby, however, could not stop crying because he didn't know whether he was Protestant, Catholic or Jewish.

THE MUGGING

It was a cold winter's evening, and my mother had gone out with her friends. I was with my Dad and a friend of mine, who was staying the night. As it was quite late my Dad did not feel like cooking, so he sent Tommy (my friend) and I to the fish and chip shop.

We walked up the cold and badly lit street, wondering whether we would get mugged. We got to the top of the street and turned the corner.

As we neared the shop we started to run, so we could get into the warmth. The chippy had three people in it, all men. The first one in the queue was skinny and had a tattoo on his right cheek. Second in line was a young man who lived in my street. He had a 'butch' figure and red hair. The last one was a small man with thick plastic-rimmed National Health glasses and bushy eyebrows.

We bought sausage and chips, and there was six pounds and one pence change left out of the ten pounds my dad had given me. We walked out of the chip shop and down to the end of my street, where I jokingly said to Tommy, 'I hope we don't get mugged.'

He laughed, but just at that moment a boy who had come up behind us said, 'Give us your money.'

'We haven't got any money,' I said.

'I saw you give a tenner to the man in the "chippy", so don't give me no trouble. Just hand over the money!'

I took out two pounds and gave it to him, but he saw that I had more money in my hand.

'Give me the rest or I'll have to beat you up,' said the boy, who was about seventeen. He took the rest of the money and ran off down my street. Tommy and I ran off towards my house. When we got there we banged on the door, and when my Dad answered we told him what had happened.

We all jumped in his car and drove around the area, hoping to catch the boy, but we did not find him.

So we then came home and ate our sausage and chips.

THE COMPUTER SHOW

We arrived at the Computer Show to find that only people over eighteen were allowed in, so we went to the organiser's office. My Dad talked to the man and he gave us a special letter saying that I had special permission from my school to go and look at things that might help with my dyslexia. They then let us into the show.

We walked into a different world, it was like the Space Control Centre in Houston. We walked down some stairs wondering where to start. I saw the Apricot stand, and said, 'Let's go there,' but we went to the IPC stand instead. However, it took us nearly half an hour to get there because my Dad kept stopping at all the stands on the way, but they had no interest for me whatsoever.

When we got to the IPC stand we had a go on the 20 Mhz Computer (Hz means how fast the computer runs, i.e. how fast a game would load.) which is five less hz than the one my Dad is getting. We could not have a go on the faster one because they had none in stock. The salesman said however that he would loan my Dad a 20Mhz machine until the faster one arrived.

We had lunch and then went to the Auto-Cad section, which is a special drawing program. You can draw in many colours, and a wide variety of shapes. I tried drawing with a mouse, and I was pushing different buttons and the computer screen went mad. It kept re-drawing St Paul's Cathedral every three seconds.

Then as the show was closing we went off to find a hotel.

The next day we had breakfast and drove off to the Exhibition Centre where we found a good parking space. We then got on to a special coach which took us to the main entrance.

We had to wait outside the entrance for half an hour, before we were let inside. We had a special map that was drawn up by a computer at the entrance to tell us where to go.

We had to find out about digitisers, laser printers, plotters and Desk Top Publishing.

A digitiser is a sort of a screen on a table, which makes it easy to draw. A laser printer is a printer which uses a laser to print letters on a page. A plotter is like a printer but is used only for drawings. It has an arm which holds pens to draw with.

My Dad's computer will also have Desk Top Publishing so he can do presentations, and he has also promised to put my stories into a book. We also looked at scanners, where you put something underneath it and it comes up on the screen. You could enlarge it and move part of it into another part.

We also saw a board which you could draw on in felt-tip pen and it would print out. Also on our walk around we saw massive monitors which were three foot wide and two foot high.

The most amazing thing I saw was the plotters. You could watch them for hours, moving in all different directions at really fast speeds. It was like watching an artist in Fast Forward, and we collected many different drawings from the different plotters.

There were lots of competitions to enter but you have to have a business card. However there was one you could enter without a card, so we did. We don't know who won yet, but we might get a letter.

I enjoyed the two days and I hope I can go to the Computer Show again next year.

THE GREAT FIGHT

There once lived a boy and his family in a small house just outside of the city. This boy loved to box, he had his own gloves, and a second-hand punch-bag, as he came from a very poor family.

Now! There was to be a fight between two great fighters, Killer Kamiller and Floppy Joe. Floppy Joe was called this because every time he fought, he always went floppy. Floppy Joe was the little boy's hero. The boy loved going to the fights, but he was so poor he could only go once a year.

But one day Floppy Joe was driving past the boy's house and saw him punching the bag. So he stopped the car and said, 'Would you like to come and watch me fight?' The boy ran inside and said to his father and mother that Floppy Joe was outside. So the boy's parents got their coats on and ran outside and got into his car. They were all very excited about driving in Joe's car.

When they arrived at the stadium everyone came out and took photos. The boy and his parents were put into the very best seats, while Floppy Joe went off and changed to get ready for the fight.

When he was announced, he did not come out, so the boy sneaked down to the changing rooms, and found Floppy Joe on the floor knocked out cold.

So the boy put on his own shorts, and Floppy Joe's gloves and went out into the ring.

The crowd cheered as the boy went into the ring, as Killer Kamiller looked down on the boy and said, 'Let's fight.'

They started fighting but Killer Kamiller was too big and kept missing. The boy punched as hard as he could, but it didn't do anything at first. However about the tenth punch Killer Kamiller started to show that he was weakening.

Then! On the 21st punch Killer Kamiller fell to the ground, and was out for the count.

Floppy Joe could not believe his eyes. He was so happy he invited the boy to come and live in his big house, and said he would train him to be a professional boxer.

So! This is what he did, and they lived happily ever after.

TWO POEMS

SQUASH

The rubber ball bounces to and fro
The aimless bodies dragging around the court
Hitting that poor defenceless ball
And then
The ball goes dead
Then it all starts again.

TIME

Time is fast
Time is slow
Time is good
Time is bad
Time is in space
Time is in the air
Time is all around
Time is Nowhere
Time is Time.

MURDER IN THE DARK

'Albert, answer the door,' said Lord Grimsby.

'Yes, my lord,' said Albert, as he opened the door and let the last of the guests in. As they walked into the cocktail room, the servants handed them drinks.

The cook, of course, was in the kitchen getting the first course ready.

The cocktail room was filled with a murmuring of voices, which would every so often get louder and then softer again.

Suddenly! The lights flickered, went off, then on, then finally off again. Everybody screamed, then, just as suddenly they were back on again. There on the floor lay the owner of the house, Lord Grimsby.

One of the guests crouched down, saying, 'Stand back, I am a doctor.' He put his hand on the lord's neck and said, 'He is dead!' A lady burst into tears, and the people said to the butler to get her to her room and to call the police.

Shortly afterwards the sound of sirens could be heard, and in walked Inspector Shy. He said, 'I would like to ask everyone some questions, so all of you must remain on the premises.'

The first to be questioned was Sir William Hawk.

'What happened?' said the inspector.

'Well!' said Sir William, 'My wife and I arrived at the house at half past seven, and we started drinking cocktails. Then at eleven o'clock, the last people came in. The lights then started flickering off and on, they went off, and when they came on again Lord Grimsby was dead.'

The inspector asked the same questions to all the guests, and they all gave similar answers.

The cook was next to be questioned. She said, 'I saw Master Jonathon go to the cellar where the main power supply is.'

The inspector then questioned Count Grimsby, Lord Grimsby's son, why he was down in the cellar. Count Grimsby denied he was there.

Inspector Shy decided to question everyone again, and they all gave the same account of their actions as last time, except the cook.

But before the inspector could arrest her, realising she had been found out, she went 'mad' and ran out of the kitchen, and up the stairs to Lady Grimsby's room, where she barricaded the door and took Lady Grimsby out on to the balcony where she held her hostage.

This lasted until the next day when she killed Lady Grimsby by stabbing her in the back of the neck with a knife steel, which was used for sharpening knives. Then she stood on the ledge of the balcony and dived four floors head first on to the drive.

JUNGLE GIRLS

The year was 1950. Lord Bellchest was taking his children on holiday to Africa. There were a lot of stopovers on the way, to pick up food and water. This story is about one of those stops.

In Zambia, where they had planned a stopover, it had taken a month to get the food, water and fuel to the makeshift airstrip in the jungle.

When the plane landed here the two girls said, 'Can we play outside?' There was a sharp 'No!', and the girls' glee faded.

Their father got up as the plane came to a halt, and as a servant opened the door of the plane, Lord Bellchest walked importantly off. 'What's this, no car!' he said.

Then came a message over the plane's radio, saying that the supplies would be late in finally arriving. The girls were then allowed off the plane, and they went off and played a game of noughts and crosses.

One of the girls suddenly spotted a lake through the trees, so they jumped up and ran over to it. They played there until they were very tired and they fell asleep. They were awakened by a shout from their Dad. Scared he would punish them, they ran off into the jungle.

Soon they found themselves lost, as they had gone off in the wrong direction. They became scared and frightened, so they looked for a sheltered place and tried to sleep.

The next day they awoke to find four black panthers staring down at them, and to their surprise they had a baby panther curled up asleep around them. ·

The eldest girl picked up the baby and put it on the ground.

'Why did you take our baby from us?' said the panther.

The eldest girl, shocked at hearing a talking panther, said, 'It came into our shelter when we were asleep, and we did not know he was there. Is he a boy?'

'Yes,' the panther replied, 'he will be our king when he is older.'

'Do you know where we are?' said the little sister.

'You are in the jungle in Zambia,' the panther replied.

'We know that! But where in the jungle?' said her sister.

'On the north side,' said one of the other panthers.

The girls then told the panthers what had happened to them, and asked if they could be taken back to their father. They agreed, and the panthers took the girls back to the south side, carrying them on their backs. They were only halfway there when a bullet came out from the trees and hit the ground, narrowly missing one of them. The panthers cringed and then froze.

Out of the trees came the girls' father with a gun in his hand, and shouted, 'Move away from the panthers so we can kill them.'

'No!' said the girls, and turned the panthers around and rode off into the jungle, never to be seen again.

THE STEALING OF THE CROWN JEWELS

On Christmas Eve the Crown Jewels were stolen.

I am an inspector and this is my account of the robbery.

There were three drunken men outside the palace at 11 pm. They proceeded to knock out the guard at the gate. As they scaled the gate the alarm was set off by the security camera. Guards were sent to apprehend the intruders.

As the guards arrived at the scene they were shot by the three men, who then threw them into the moat. The three men then went up to the security guards' rooms and shot the guards in the room.

By this time the alarm had been raised and police were already on the scene. From the guard room, the men carried on up towards the vault, shooting the guards as they went. One of the three intruders was shot by pursuing policemen as they neared the main vault.

At the vault they placed dynamite at the entrance, and the following blast blew open the door and killed two of the policemen. The men grabbed the Crown Jewels, and climbed to the top of the palace where a Microlight picked them up and took them to a private airfield.

Here they stole an air force jet and flew it to a jungle landing strip in Mali in Africa. The jet was followed there, by the SAS, but the criminals managed to escape into the jungle and are still being 'pursued'.

We have found out that the three men (one of them may have been a woman) killed ten guards and wounded four others.

These men will be captured and brought back 'Dead or Alive'.

Signed

Inspector Paris Innes

THE TIMES

April 1st 1995

THE CROWN JEWELS STOLEN
BY ARMED GANG

We have just discovered the names of the gang in the recent theft of the Crown Jewels from the palace. Their names are Fred, Bob and their Mum, Hilda. The two men were dustbin men from Chelsea.

The man who flew the plane was Prince Charles, and Princess Di flew the Microlight.

In a press release the next day Margaret Thatcher said, 'I knew that the royal family could not be trusted, so I have placed them in the London Dungeon, and next Thursday my coronation will be held at Westminster Abbey!'

Other News

Rupert Murdoch has become Chancellor of the Exchequer, when in an overwhelming vote 27 million *Sun* readers made this a requirement for the newly elected government.

The pound slips to an all-time low against the Polish 'Zlote', and the American 'Yen'.

THE CLOCK

In my house there used to be a clock. It was hand painted with two naked babies on the sides, both holding flaming torches. The old clock ticked away for 150 years until one day it stopped.

We were a poor family, living in a draughty old house in the countryside, so we were not able to take it to the clockmenders because it would have cost too much to have it fixed.

When the clock stopped strange things started happening to my family. At first we thought it was just bad luck, just things going wrong as they sometimes do. First the car wouldn't start and then the phone went dead. However, when we went to check the wires they had been cut.

This made us think that something weird was going on so my Dad got his gun out of the cabinet and loaded it.

Frightened, we all went into the sitting room. That was the worst thing we could have done, but we didn't know that until it was too late!

It was the *clock*!

The first of my family to get killed was my Dad because he was the nearest to the clock. One of its doors opened and a hand came out and started to slowly strangle him. The only one who saw the hand coming was my little sister, but she was deaf and dumb and was unable to warn him. As he died, he was dragged into the clock.

My mother grabbed the gun and shot at the hand. It missed and the hand got away into the clock. My mother sat there, holding the gun in the air, ready to shoot.

After a while, though, we all fell asleep, which I now realise was due to the clock. I was awoken by my mother screaming. When I looked, the naked babies were burning into her back.

I shouted, 'No.'

The babies looked around. I kicked them off, grabbed the gun and fired!

I got one, and its remains spread across the wall.

I then pulled my mother and sister up and we ran to the door. It was locked! We ran upstairs to my bedroom where we stayed, until we heard crashing from downstairs. I went down to investigate.

The clock had light coming out of it, then it transformed into a green monster with red eyes and long sharp nails. I ran out to where it could see me, and fired my remaining shots. Then I ran up the stairs to my bedroom, but my mother and sister had gone.

I saw them running away from the house through my window. I went to climb out of my window, but it slammed shut. I turned and there, was the green monster.

I said, 'Why did you let my family go, and not me?'

The green monster said, 'Because *you* are the one I want.'

Then he reached down and plunged his claw through my body. My eyes saw red, then black and then I was in Heaven.

'It is nice here as everything is good. There is no Evil and no monsters.'

'That is all I want to say to you, Mum.'

Love Paris.

From Heaven.

DEMON DAMIEN

CHAPTER 1
THE BOY

This is a story about a boy called Damien, who had no home, no family, nothing, and was always in trouble. He did, however, go to school as he liked it, even though he didn't attend lessons. What he did like was reading and sport.

He had blond scruffy hair, blue eyes and ripped clothes. He had one thing special about him. No little finger on his left hand as it had been bitten off by his father who had gone crazy.

Each day he had a social worker come around to the park where he lived and slept. On this particular day the social worker came with two men. He overheard one of the men saying to his social worker, 'Where does he normally sleep?' The social worker pointed towards him. He turned and started to run, but as he ran through some thick undergrowth something grabbed him by the hair and pulled him up into the air to a cloud.

CHAPTER 2
DEMON meets DAMIEN

As he landed in the cloud, a three-foot-high man stood in front of him. He was wearing glasses and a dustman's cap.

To Damien's amazement he started to talk.

'Hello I'm Vass, I'm a Demon from Qil.'

'Thank you for saving me from those men. My name is Damien,' said the boy.

The demon turned his head to one side and then back again. Damien stared at the little man and said, 'How did you pull me up as you are so small?'

'You forget I am a demon, I can do most things,' said Vass.

'Can you take me back down, because I am scared of heights?' Damien asked.

The cloud slowly sunk to the ground, faded away, and the two of them started to walk through the park. They talked about each other's lives, especially about Qil and what it was like to live there.

Vass told Damien how he had been deported because he didn't like the way the leader was running Qil. The demon then asked Damien to join him to stop what was happening in Qil. Damien said that he would try.

That night Damien went with the Demon to Stonehenge where he lay down a great carpet and sat on it.

CHAPTER 3
RITUALS

After Vass had laid down the carpet and sat on it he asked Damien to join him. Damien started to walk towards the carpet, but as he got nearer, he felt himself being gently lifted into the air and then put down again on the carpet. He sat down and then the demon mumbled some words. Instantly there was a flash of green light, and a voice which shouted, 'Ifto dgde ewq hafte' (a Qilian dialect).

He then found himself being pulled into the demon's body. When he looked it was from the demon's eyes, and he saw that he had disappeared. Then from deep inside Vass's body he heard himself say to the demon, 'Can we change into my body?'

Vass said, 'Yes, we can change into anything we want.'

Damien then felt himself being pulled out from within the demon and with another flash of green light he was back to his normal self. But not quite! He suddenly realised that this time the demon was inside him.

Damien felt himself lifting from the ground and up into the cloud again where it took him back to the park. Here in a special marquee there was a Paranormal Professors' Convention taking place.

The cloud landed and Damien mysteriously appeared, just as the convention was being opened. Unluckily for them, a professor saw it happen, and alerted the others.

That's when they began the chase.

CHAPTER 4
TROUBLE COMES

The boy started to run when he saw the professors chasing after him. He heard the demon's voice inside him telling him that he should use his powers to stop them.

He stopped, turned around, and faced his pursuers. The professors all stopped, and then proceeded cautiously towards the boy.

Damien waved his hands and suddenly all the trees around them came crashing down.

Damien turned to run, but he heard a snapping noise and felt a searing pain. He looked down and there was an animal trap caught on his foot. Before he could release himself a man grabbed him from behind, pulling him into the bushes. The man then dragged him through some trees, along a footpath, and then across a road to a house.

It was a small house with dark curtains and drab furniture. Once inside the house he was put into a room with potions bubbling and bunsen burners burning. Then he was put in a cage and the trap was removed.

Suddenly he felt a pain all through his body and then he screamed. The man who had been working with the potions stood up and Damien saw his distorted face for the first time. It was dark skinned with scratch marks down it.

Damien knew the face. It was the face of a mad scientist who had gone crazy when a snake had bitten him, and he was never the same again.

He was wearing a black cloak and dark blue jeans, and he had a smile on his face. He started to speak in a gruff voice.

'Who are you and where do you come from?'

'I am Damien and I come from New York.'

'Don't lie. I too saw you come from the sky in that cloud,' said the mad scientist.

'No, I didn't come from the sky, you must have been imagining it,' Damien replied.

'Well, I will find out sooner or later,' said the mad scientist.

'How will you find out?' asked Damien.

'By shooting you, of course,' replied the mad scientist.

'No, don't shoot me! *Please*! I didn't fly from the sky, *please*!'

The man walked across the room, picked up a shot gun, turned, and fired. The shot sped across the room and hit Damien. He felt a sharp pain in the chest and as his vision blurred, he fell and the cage exploded.

'I knew it! I knew it!' the mad scientist shouted.

A blinding light came from Damien's mouth and the scientist went flying backwards and was killed. Damien found himself being taken out through the skylight in the roof and floating off.

CHAPTER 5
DEATH

Damien landed in an alley way where he became aware of the demon's voice. It said, 'I must come out of your body so you can live and I shall take the bullet and die.'

'No, let me die, and you can live and save your people,' pleaded Damien.

'That is OK. You shall receive my powers and you can save my people,' replied Vass.

'You should save your people, not me,' said Damien.

'My mind is made up, I have started the process,' replied Vass.

Damien once again felt great pain in his chest, and then his injuries went away. Then he saw the demon on the floor with green blood coming out of him.

Damien picked up the demon and started to run with him. He ran and ran until he got to the park, where the demon died, at the same spot where they had first met.

The boy buried him there and walked away into the trees.

To this day no one knows what happened to Damien. We think however he saved Qil, but some say he still lives in the park, but no-one really knows.

OUR EXPERIENCES AS THE PARENTS OF A DYSLEXIC CHILD

by TREVOR and MAGGIE INNES

Just the sound of the word dyslexia conjures images of some fatal disease.

This section is intended to relate our experience of dyslexia as it manifested itself through Paris. The frustration we felt as parents led us to try to help him ourselves, and so far this has made an amazing difference to his ability to write and express himself.

We hope that our experience may be of benefit or at least offer hope to the thousands of children who are classed as having 'specific learning difficulties'. This new terminology does not disguise the fact that these children often see themselves as stupid. Many dyslexics have high IQs, but they have a problem in the area of hand-eye co-ordination which affects their ability to produce decent-looking written work.

The word dyslexia comes from two Greek words, *dus* meaning diseased, abnormal or difficult and *legein*, to speak. The dictionary definition is 'impaired ability to read (not caused by low intelligence)'.

How do you tell if your child is dyslexic?

This is very difficult to assess, especially at an early age. Until Paris was six, when he finished his first year at school, he didn't seem to have any real problems. He was quite a chirpy sort, happy-go-lucky and very chatty. He had his moodies, but we took that as being pretty normal.

In fact, throughout his first four years of school, we were always told that he was average and OK. There can be a huge variation in the abilities of young children and the point at which they start learning. We were frequently told he was just a late developer.

At the time there was a lot of talk in the media about the effects of lead on children, and naturally we were worried that this might be Paris's problem. Of course, it turned out to be nothing of the sort.

I think the first time anyone mentioned that there was anything wrong was one term when he had a supply teacher fresh from college, who noticed that he was second from bottom in his class in maths, but was obviously much brighter than this suggested. The 'accentuating the positive' approach which is common in schools nowadays can be quite destructive, because it can hide real problems.

One of the difficulties about diagnosing dyslexia is that there are varying degrees of severity, and a wide range of specific symptoms. One of the signs in younger children is a difficulty in kicking or catching a ball, which Paris had no problems with at all; on the other hand, many dyslexics fail at writing but are good at maths, which Paris certainly wasn't. All this makes it very hard to assess.

Here is a list of the more common signs of dyslexia; if four or five of these pointers apply to your child, it may be time to do something about it.

1 Writing Bs, Ds and Ps back to front.

2 Mixing numbers or columns, as in writing 67 instead of 76. 6s and 9s reversed, or written in mirror image are also typical. In columns Paris still quite often adds up the hundreds first, and has worked out his own immensely complicated method of addition, to try to cope. Although many people object strongly to children using calculators from an early age, it may be the only answer. It is for Paris.

3 Confusion between left and right.

4 Confusion about days, months and the time from a conventional clock face, although a digital clock seems to present no problems.

5 Spelling difficulties. These can be very severe as you can see from the examples of Paris's writing at the back of the book: he wrote these after two years' specialist help and tuition. The problems include leaving letters out, putting letters in the wrong order, and writing the wrong words (confusing by, buy and bye; father and farther, etc).

6 Great difficulty with the physical process of writing.

7 Inaccurate reading, with poor comprehension and often a real reluctance to read at all. Skipping questions in a test, or lines in reading.

8 Low self-esteem and self-confidence. A tendency to think he or she is stupid, despite showing obvious intelligence in other ways.

9 The opposite of the above, claiming to be able to do things he or she obviously can't.

10 Taking much longer than the average to complete written tasks, and requiring immense concentration for little result.

11 Cross co-ordination. Everyone has one arm, leg, eye, etc stronger than the other. Paris is right-eared, right-handed, right-legged, but left-eyed.

12 Aggressive or disruptive behaviour.

13 Inconsistency in work. A friend of ours was bottom of the class in English, but top in maths.

14 Building up a defence mechanism against criticism and resentment to being helped. Oversensitivity, with all criticism taken to heart, as it seems they are always wrong.

15 A history of ear infections when younger.

16 Bed-wetting, possibly a sign of frustration.

17 Becoming a master of deception, going to enormous lengths to hide the problem so as not to be considered stupid.

Estimates of the numbers of people suffering from dyslexia suggest that at least 4% of the population have such problems, which represents over 2 million people in Britain alone. This means that there are an estimated 350,000 dyslexic schoolchildren or, on average, at least one in every classroom in the country.

Unfortunately, while individual schools recognise the problem, much of the education system does not, and even if it did the problem is so great that there are no resources in state schools to provide the intensive teaching needed. There are many more resources available in private education, including several schools specifically for the dyslexic. Classes are much smaller, and teaching is sometimes even done on a one to one basis, but this can cost up to £250 a week, more than most people can afford.

There are now several specialist centres for dyslexia where you can send your child for a couple of hours' extra tuition at least twice a week (this seems to be the minimum required). But this will only be of use if they can fit you in, as places are always in great demand; if you live within reasonable travelling distance; and if you can afford the £10–15 per hour, twice a week.

Few teachers have been taught how to recognise dyslexia, or what to do about it when they do. Children who find they cannot learn no matter how hard they try simply lose interest. They become disruptive and insolent or play truant. One troublesome pupil can disturb the whole class, so nobody gets any work done.

We have found a way to solve the problem, at least for Paris; other people with similar difficulties who have tried the same methods have also found the results very encouraging. But it is not an easy route. The child needs great self-discipline, or a strong-willed parent who is able to put up with a lot of verbal flak along the lines of 'Do I have to?' 'No one else gets any homework, why should I have to do it?' 'I hate you!' etc. This can also be accompanied by the banging of doors. An introverted child might not express resentment this way, but you can be sure he or she is thinking something like it.

Within the state system, there are large numbers of potentially very good schools which now find that all their resources are used just to keep the school running, and nothing is left over to cope with special needs students.

Although Paris's school suffers from some of these problems, it would not have been possible to write this book or achieve what we have without its help, and especially the help of Paris's head of year. Without her insight, her willingness to let us try and solve problems for ourselves and finding time to fit us into her already heavy workload, we would still be at square one. Many schools would simply have said it was impossible and dismissed us.

To my mind, there are several problems in the current education system, which severely affect the chances of dyslexic children ever reaching their full potential.

In today's changing job market, where manual and unskilled work is often done by machine, it is more than ever important for school leavers to be able to spell and write coherently. Dyslexic children are often very bright, and the technology exists to help them get round their problem – they could contribute an enormous amount to the future of the country if only the resources were available to teach them.

It can be extremely difficult to assess the standard of the school to which you send your child if overall results are given in percentages. '67% passed maths' may sound fine, but if, for example, 50% got an F grade and 17% an E grade, the standard would have been pretty poor.

In the first three years of some secondary schools, there are no guidelines to tell parents what the children should achieve at the end of each year, to give them some indication of how well they will eventually do in their GCSE exams. As far as we can find out, these guidelines do exist, but by no means all schools give them out. With luck the National Curriculum will eventually attend to this, but many students from different schools have said to us that when the fourth year and the start of the GCSEs come along, they find themselves so far behind they are unable to catch up.

There is a fine line to be drawn here, as many parents are unrealistic about what their child can achieve. Too much pressure to achieve can be just as destructive as lack of concern. This is true of all children, but the additional difficulty with dyslexia is that the root problem of communication has to be solved before achievement can start. And it should be said that parental apathy is one of the worst problems that any child, dyslexic or not, can have to combat.

The argument against a structured guideline is that it will put off the less able students. Our experience has been that without any structure or idea of what they are learning and any sort of reason for doing so, many students feel there is no point in learning at all. This is especially true of dyslexic children, who often find they are putting in enormous effort for little result anyway.

In many schools, textbooks are virtually abandoned. Instead, students are given photocopied sheets of paper – the most expensive way of producing a document in the numbers required. These papers often get lost or crumpled, and the degree of organisation required to keep them in some vestige of order would be beyond most adults.

Without books, students cannot look back at what they have done or what they need to achieve for the future. For revision, they only have their own notes. Again, what is already difficult for normal children may pose insurmountable problems for dyslexics.

Many parents who want to help, but whose education did not encompass much of the technology now being used and taught in schools, are lost; and with no textbooks or outlines of what their children are trying to achieve, they feel even more helpless if their child's problems are complicated by dyslexia.

One argument that was put to me by a head of department (not from Paris's school) was that, with money so short in state schools, parents should buy textbooks. This happens in many countries round the world and has the advantage that children are more inclined to take care of property if they have their parents to answer to. Books would be provided for those who could not afford to buy them. It is certainly easier for teachers to use textbooks, and they have not been abandoned from choice.

At the very least, surely parents should be given each year a list of books that are used by the school, which they could buy if they chose. This list should also include books to help dyslexics and children with other specific learning difficulties. The biggest resource that the system has to help it at the moment, in the time of acute shortages, is the parents.

Another trend in some secondary schools is not to mark pupils' class work or homework in the first three years. The idea seems to be that if the work is marked with a percentage or a grade, it discourages students who have not done well. This may be true, but unless some sort of structure exists, how does anyone know how well or badly they are doing? Dyslexic children often become disruptive if they find they are getting nowhere however hard they try – what chance do they have if they have no feedback or encouragement?

There are two basic systems of education – mixed ability and streamed. Mixed ability works well when there are plenty of resources, *true* mixed ability classes, not those with an unbalanced intake, small classes and back-up when problems arise. Because of shortages, this is becoming impossible.

The Cockcroft report (an extensive report into the teaching of maths, published in 1982) has shown that in any single class there can be as much as a seven year learning difference between the students. In other words, at the age of 11, some children cannot do the work of a seven-year-old and some can easily do the work of a 14-year-old. With such a wide range of abilities, the problem of diagnosing dyslexia within a large class becomes even more difficult.

Streaming poses different problems. If the school has its streaming right the difference in ability between students in any one class is cut drastically, and this should help reduce the enormous burden on teachers. But it spells disaster for dyslexic children, as they are then grouped with the lowest ability. By the nature of their problem, they tend to be disruptive, so that when they are all grouped together the result can be virtually unteachable classes. This may help the rest of the school keep its standards high, but it is essentially the end of an education for a dyslexic child.

Probably the most dramatic problem of all lies in the teaching of English. Punctuation, spelling and grammar are 'no longer considered important' in many schools. But the readability of the students' written exam paper is what determines their exam results: they have to put their thoughts and knowledge on paper logically and coherently, and the examiner has to be able to read what they write. As you will see from the examples at the back of the book, this

91

can make the difference between a good grade and a fail. It's like looking at work done by two different people, which in a sense it is.

The phonetic teaching of English has been replaced by the 'look and learn' method. The problem is that large numbers of students benefit from both systems, yet you can only have one, and the 'look and learn' method simply does not work for children with dyslexia and other learning problems.

I was taught the phonetic way, and the advantages are really being brought home to me as I write this: if I don't know how to spell a word, I can sound it out phonetically and get it correct or within the spell-checker's range of abilities. But without this method, unless you have memorised a word, you really have no idea how to spell it. Of course, it does not work for every word, but it does for a large number.

What the phonetic system does is give you an extra tool for reading optically-stored information which may have got a little jumbled in the storage process, or may never have been stored properly in the first place.

The way a subject is taught can probably make as much difference as anything in the teaching of dyslexic children. Many subjects are taught in a way that is completely abstract, not applied or practical, with no reference to material objects or specific examples. This makes them particularly hard to understand. For Paris this has especially applied to English and maths, probably the two most important subjects. (In English, to be fair, the literary side is fine, but the writing of it, the structure of the language and the ability to write it has been lost.) Most of the other subjects seem much better. Although the problem is severe at the moment, things are changing rapidly and more practical alternatives are available if you know where to look and what to look for.

There is a fine balance between positive and negative thinking.

One of the main do's of dyslexia for parents is always to stress the things the child is good at. But no matter how much you stress a dyslexic child's positive attributes, dyslexia will not go away, and there comes a time when its problems become paramount. This is also true in the school environment, which was the main reason we decided something had to be done.

Paris's school report for the last term of 1988 stressed only the positive, saying that he didn't have any real problems, was about average and doing OK generally. We later discovered that 'average' meant an exam result F, which in the current system is just scraping a pass – we, and lots of other parents we've spoken to, always assumed that 'average' was a C grade.

That report really rang alarm bells, as we knew Paris's reading and writing were absolutely appalling. He knew it, too, which compounded his problems. What he wrote was gibberish much of the time – to us and to his teachers. It was not their fault, they were not experts on dyslexia, but the philosophy of always stressing the positive was hiding the reality.

Paris's school psychologist, who has since been promoted, was responsible for the children with learning difficulties, of which dyslexia was one of many, for over 30 schools (at the time there was an unfilled vacancy, and she had to double her workload).

Many parents have expressed anger to us about the educational psychologist's lack of response to their needs. The truth of the matter is that to become an educational psychologist requires a five or six year university degree followed by two years' teaching before you can practise. So there is never going to be an abundance of them. They are responsible for the whole range of 'special needs', of which dyslexia is but a part: educational psychologists are responsible for the partially sighted and the blind; for the deaf – those with permanent or temporary hearing loss; for the dumb; for those with behavioural problems which may be the result of social deprivation, sexual or physical abuse; and for those with any one of the multiplicity of other problems such as sensory learning difficulties, autism, Down's syndrome, cerebral palsy and many other difficulties or handicaps.

You can see the problem the dyslexic child has in terms of priorities. He or she may be lucky to be seen once or twice a year. Paris's school has three special needs teachers for 1500 students. Given that an estimated 4% of the population have dyslexic problems, that means there are 60 dyslexic students in the school, let alone the myriad other learning problems that have to be dealt with. So basically, as parents, you are on your own, which is why we have had to take the practical approach we have to Paris's difficulties.

Being the parent of a dyslexic child is probably similar to being the parent of any other child with a physical or mental disability, but with the added problem that dyslexia is intangible and difficult to recognise. As there are few clear or even consistent outward signs, it can be a long time before it is seen that dyslexia is the problem, and it might only be by chance that the problem is recognised and given a name.

As a result, parents and child experience feelings of real frustration and helplessness, as both are aware that there is a major problem, but don't know what it is. Parents don't know where to begin to help. People who have learned to read and write without difficulty have no concept of what's troubling their child.

Pick up a complicated textbook on a topic of which you know nothing, like computer programming: it's really like reading a foreign language, even though it's written in English. Or imagine that you are trying to write a computer program: you follow the instructions to the letter, it doesn't work and no matter how hard you try you can't make it work. Then you find that all that is missing is an *. This will give you an idea of what dyslexics are up against.

The written word was our biggest nightmare and we felt completely helpless until the portable word processor came along. It has made at least an 80% improvement in Paris's ability to communicate on paper, and it has raised his self esteem and confidence beyond his wildest dreams.

Our efforts seem to indicate that the brain can recognise words when they come up on a word-processor screen, and tell if they are correctly spelt, whereas it could not do this if they were hand-written. This seems to happen 60% of the time – that is, just using the word processor seems to eliminate 60% of the mistakes he would have made otherwise – with another 30% of words being identified as wrong by the 'Spell-Right' dictionary. The problem we can find no way round for the moment, is that of the remaining 10% – wrong words in a sentence, spelled correctly but wrong in context. However, give the boffins another few years and they may well find a way of checking that the word is right in context as well.

When you are writing, your brain has to visualise the individual letters, join them mentally into words and sentences, and then transmit messages to your arm, wrist, hand and fingers, so that they can join all the letters together legibly, keep an even spacing between the words, maintain a uniform height of the letters, calculate the line length to get the last word as close to the right hand margin as possible, move back to the left hand side of the page and down the correct distance to the next line.

Someone with severe dyslexia has to do all this laboriously for each letter and word, which is why it becomes very hard work. To make matters worse, you have very little to show for an immense amount of effort. Paris's description of this is that it's like a nerve gone wrong inside, between his brain and his hand, and no matter how hard he tries, his pen will not do what he tells it to.

This is where the word processor comes into its own, because it performs most of these functions for you. All you need to know is where the keys are located, and with training this becomes automatic, as writing is for most people. Of course, the greatest advantage is that when you make a mistake, corrections are easy and you can edit out anything you don't like without making your work untidy.

The other major advantage is having a 90,000 word dictionary and thesaurus at your fingertips. This makes the conventional dictionary redundant, except for looking up meanings.

Work which used to be impossible to read can now be as good as the child's abilities permit, with the exception that if dyslexia was discovered late and a child fell behind at school, he or she may still have some catching up to do before attaining their 'natural' level. They still have to work harder than most children, and still get exhausted, but it will not be as bad as it used to be. As the results of their labour will be neat and easy to read, it will give them a sense of achievement.

The best system we have found so far is the Smith Corona PWP 7000, which is a small compact lap top word processor, light and small enough to be put in a bag or backpack. It comes with a letter quality printer which Paris uses to print his day's work out at home. It has been Paris's salvation and after six weeks' concentrated effort, it made more difference than two and a half years of specialist help.

The secret ingredient that makes this particular machine brilliant is its 'Spell-Right' dictionary, which bleeps at you when you make a mistake. You can access the dictionary in three different ways to find the correct spelling for a word, and this program seems to be much better at picking up phonetic mistakes than others we have tried.

The Smith Corona PWP 7000 only came out in November 1989; before that we had the PWP60, which did the same job but needed a power point in the classroom (the 7000 is both battery and mains operated). The only power point in one of Paris's classrooms, in which he frequently used his word processor, stopped working, and it took the school five months to fix it. So we needed a truly portable alternative, and found the PWP 7000.

Another point is that it is a serious business machine, not a games one, and in fact it's one on which you can't play games. This puts a whole different light on the reason for using it. Psychologically, a computer on which you can play games always has the temptation there. The portable doesn't have this temptation, so when you are using it, your approach is much more professional. It's there for you to do your work, period.

The Japanese are planning to install ten million computers in their schools over the next ten years. This has been made possible by the extraordinary developments in computer chip technology – a machine that can compute one million instructions per second would have cost about £31,000 in 1981 and costs £300 in 1990. This says a lot about what education is going to be like in the future.

To get Paris up and running, we spent an hour a day together for 25 days, learning how the word processor worked and trying to master a new function each day, because we were both computer illiterates. After that we made him sit down for an hour each evening and, if he had no homework, he would write a story of his choice, which is how this book came into being.

He used to moan quite a lot about this at first, then suddenly he would have an idea for a story and he would sit down and out it would come, flowing into the portable word processor as it never could by hand. Although he had had ideas before, it was a huge relief to him to be able to express himself so that others could read what he had written.

After he had written about 35 stories, we realised that it would make an excellent little book, so we put it together and produced 60 copies to give to friends and family as Christmas presents.

It should be said here that our experience may not work for everyone, although I think that the two disciplines of typing and learning the portable word processor will together give a dyslexic child the greatest assistance, for the least possible cost in the long term. A combination of this and specialist help would be ideal.

Paris has never really been able to get into reading, and still has problems understanding what he has read. Yet his vocabulary has always been very good. The only books he has ever really enjoyed are those by Roald Dahl, and the 'Asterix' series. Roald Dahl certainly fired his imagination and Asterix and Obelix also gave him a good grounding in the understanding of people and places, as these books are brilliant in their observations of different cultures and customs. The 'Asterix' books have two other advantages: they are written in cartoon strip format, which means every bit of text has an illustration to go with it, which helps make the meaning clearer; and the text is written in block capitals, which Paris finds easier to read.

He had remedial reading help from the age of eight, but it didn't help much until he started the phonetic way of sounding out his words; then he did make some progress. But even now he finds it very laborious and would never read for pleasure or relaxation.

Once again, technology has provided a partial solution. The cassette recorder has been a saving grace, and Paris still falls asleep listening to a story tape. This means that if you can get the books you want on tape (and there are lots available), your child can still have the pleasure of listening to good stories; it is also an enormous help with vocabulary, pronunciation and sentence construction. Children can learn to express themselves well orally, even if they have severe reading and writing difficulties. Several of Paris's tapes, particularly the Asterix ones and *The Secret Diary of Adrian Mole*, are nearly worn out.

One of the main problems we had to solve in the school environment was the logistics of using a word processor in a system that is just not set up for it. Security, a place to charge it up overnight, and the lack of power points have all had to be dealt with. Lessons tend to be spread around the school, so we had to find somewhere to store the word processor at lunchtime. We have just had our first machine stolen after 15 months. It is now Paris's lifeline to literacy, so we have no choice but to get him another. If it happens again, I don't know what we will do. The battery portable has given the biggest single boost to his abilities, but this also makes it more portable for the thieves.

We have wondered many times whether we are doing the right thing in taking Paris's problems into our own hands, but the results so far have surpassed anything we could have hoped for. This is especially true of the major obstacles of English and maths.

After struggling for two and a half years with the abstract maths taught in Paris's school and doing the best we could to help, we were getting nowhere. What we needed was a system of teaching maths in an everyday context, so that he could see some point to what he was learning. It would have to be written in a way he could understand and be practical enough to be of some benefit to him in life, even if his exam results were not brilliant.

Heinemann Educational Books produce three textbooks called *Foundation Maths*, *Central Maths* and *Challenging Maths*, for the three different levels of maths examination. They all teach maths in terms of everyday life: problems may be about planning your kitchen, going on holiday, interest rates, income tax and so on. So the maths has a context and provides a reference book for things that will be useful in real life. Writing maths is still a problem for Paris, but if we can solve this, we will have coped with most of his writing difficulties.

For English, after failing to get help in punctuation, grammar, sentence forming, etc, from the school, we went out looking. We searched and searched through the unbelievable complexity of a lot of grammar books until we found *Meanings into Words*, which is published by the Cambridge University Press and is designed as a course for teaching English to non-English speakers.

When you think about it, it's the obvious place to start, if you want to learn English. The beauty of it is that it isn't in the least bit heavy, but teaches through everyday conversations and situations.

It is on three levels, intermediate, upper intermediate and proficiency, the last two corresponding to the GCSE and A level standards, and in fact it is recognised in more countries than GCSEs. The only snag is that you can't sit the exam unless English is a foreign language and you live in a non-English-speaking country. Even so, it's brilliant at teaching people how to write and makes an excellent addition to the English course.

Another two books which are concise and to the point are the Longman English Guides, *Grammar* by S.H. Burton and *Punctuation* by Ian Gordon.

Because the education system is not geared up to cope with dyslexia, we have been forced to work out practical solutions to problems with no clearcut answers. Our philosophy throughout has been 'What can we do to help?' and 'What skills can we give Paris that will enable him to get a good job?' Here are some practical things you can do.

1. Lobby your MP, local authority and the Department of Education to have dyslexia recognised and to provide the resources to deal with it.

2. Teach your child to touch type. We recommend the Smith

Corona 7000 series portable word processor as the most practical machine, as to date it is the only one with the patented 'Spell-Right/Autospell' feature, which corrects your mistakes as you make them.

3. Make sure he or she learns to use the word processor and all its functions properly.

4. If things you do to help don't work, do not give up. If it is obvious there is something the child cannot do, look for an alternative. The technology to help is available, and jobs for our children will lie in that area anyway. In the end, it may be to their advantage. For us it is still a continuous learning process and several things have emerged simply from writing this book.

5. It is still important to try and encourage the child to read, using the talking books as back-up. Before Paris had his PWP, much of his written work was gobbledygook to us with no punctuation or speech. Yet he could read it out word perfect with all the inflections of speech, despite the fact that many of the words he had written were the wrong ones: he might write 'no' when he meant 'now' or 'know'. But he would only read well if he was reading something he had written himself; if he read aloud from a book, he might well miss out on the context because of the concentration required for reading the words.

If your child's dyslexia is particularly severe, the tape recorder can help, as a teacher friend of ours found. She had to read into it for one of her pupils, and although it didn't help his literacy, and there were problems with other disruptive children reading into it, it built up his confidence and showed that he understood his subject.

6. If there is a dyslexic centre in your area, and you can afford the tuition, it is well worth while. They have helped many thousands of people, especially those whose problems are not as severe as Paris's.

7. The question of the way subjects are taught is something you will

101

have to research at your own school. If there is a problem, you can only hope the school will respond in a positive way, as Paris's school has done. But if large numbers of students need help, things may become very complicated. Major restructuring of the school's teaching system may be needed, and this might take a long time to be implemented.

If you want books to supplement what your child is being taught, you will have to search through the available material to see what will best suit your child – ideally with the help of his or her teachers. We can only advise on what has worked for us. Try to adopt a realistic attitude towards what you expect your child to achieve and what you expect from the school.

8. Under the provisions of the Education Act of 1981, if your child is severely dyslexic, you can have him or her statemented. This may provide additional teaching or equipment, depending on what the Education Authority feels is appropriate.

Concessions can also be sought from the Examinations Board, provided that the application – which must be done through the school – is supported by an educational psychologist in the six months preceding the exam, and that the dyslexia has been previously documented, the earlier the better.

The concessions may allow for the examination paper to be read to the candidate, or for some extra time for the completion of the paper. More rarely, they may allow for the use of somebody to write down the candidate's verbal responses. However, any certificate granted may be marked that the exam was taken with concessions, so you have to decide what is best for your child.

Many parents are worried about the stigma of having their child associated with an 'educational psychologist'. But there are no implications of mental illness: the educational psychologist is a trained and experienced teacher with a degree in psychology and a lot of experience in normal child development.

9. Experiment with colours. Go to your local print shop and get them to print something out on all the different coloured card they have and see which one your child finds easiest to use. Then ask the school if their sheets can be produced on that colour.

Don't be influenced by the colour *you* think is best. Paris found the black printing on a dark blue card the easiest to read, and for me it was one of the hardest. He said that all the others were very glary, and although the glary ones were easier to read at a distance, when you got within normal reading distance the darker one was much better.

We tried using different coloured acetate sheets when reading, but Paris did not find this helped him much. He also totally rebelled against the idea of coloured glasses, which for a teenage boy with enough problems as it is, is understandable.

The best solution is called inverse video, which means white lettering on a mid-grey background or similar combination of colours. This is a very efficient answer to the readability problem, because letters and words stand out on the page and the spaces then divide up the words. Normal black-on-white printing, to quote Paris, just looks like a page with lines on it.

This is why if you have the right kind of computer screen, it transforms the text's readability. Unfortunately it is a little much to ask the world's printing enterprises to change the established system, so we have to do what we can to work around it.

10. Don't let the child use dyslexia as an excuse for laziness. Be firm, but supportive and understanding. Remember that a dyslexic child has to work very hard at reading and writing, and even so may not attain great results.

11. Don't blame teachers or schools for not assessing or helping to solve the problems. Very few have specialist knowledge of dyslexia, so you will have to make them aware of what they should be looking for, and what they can do to help. But remember that dyslexia is still not a recognised problem, and they may be going out on a limb to help you.

12. If you know of other dyslexic children at your child's school, the special needs teacher may be willing to give extra lessons after school. An ideal size for the class would be three to five, so parents of all the children could share the cost (likely to be about £15 an hour). Now that local authorities are in charge of schools, this should be easier than it would have been under the previous system.

Some dyslexic centres have special assisted places for tuition, but they are few and far between. Still, if you are unemployed or have serious financial difficulties, it is worth asking.

13. Your worst enemy is time. I need at least 48 hours in a day to get through what I want to do. The best thing is to get your child to sit down for half an hour when he or she is younger, then one to two hours, every day if possible, including weekends. It still gives them plenty of time at weekends and in the evenings to do what they want to – though they may not see it like that! In this time they should do homework, read, learn the word processor, but not play computer games. If there is no homework, courses which can be done at home, such as the *Alpha to Omega* teaching book for younger children and *Meanings into Words* for older ones will prove invaluable. Although in many cases imposing this discipline is extremely difficult, nigh impossible, a dyslexic child needs this sort of determination if he or she is to do well in GCSE exams.

14. It is particularly important that the dyslexic child *wants* to overcome his or her disability, otherwise it is a waste of everyone's time. If the problem is not diagnosed early, the child may have given up all hope of an education, and there may be nothing you can do.

This book is by no means an answer to the problem of dyslexia, but we hope it shows what dyslexia is and the disastrous effects it can have on children. We have tried to show, from our own experience, what you are up against as the parents of a dyslexic child, and the solutions we have found. But there are no instant miracle cures! It requires great determination and continuous effort – but where Paris is concerned we feel it has been well worth it.

MY FIGHT AGAINST DYSLEXIA

by RICK FULLER

(Rick Fuller is a friend of our family who found that he was dyslexic before the word became commonplace. He knew he was not stupid, although his teachers and elders disagreed. He got to the top of his profession with will and determination.)

My main complaint about being dyslexic is that, like having mild asthma, it meant that I did not appreciate school as much as I should have. However, without both I probably would not be where I am now. Both conditions are similar in some ways, as both are under-diagnosed and cause the sufferer to be incorrectly labelled as unintelligent or lazy. Likewise, both can be coped with once diagnosed.

Unlike most people, I knew that I was not stupid and it amazes me now how much importance was placed on spelling. It would seem obvious that a child who is top in maths and never lower than half way down the class is not stupid, even if they can't spell. I therefore had to learn to defend myself. At primary school I became a joker and perhaps a bully. Though I was never a big success at the latter, being the former certainly helped my lecturing career. The next ploy was illness, which helped me avoid most spelling tests and reading aloud in class (the pits) but I still ended up on detention most weeks and failed the 11-plus exam, which was crucial to the rest of your schooling in those days.

Failing the 11-plus was a good thing as it kept me from traditional schools and got me to one where I was able to use my next trick, which was dropping subjects. I ruthlessly avoided all subjects which required essay-writing, so I unwittingly became a scientist. Little did I know then how much writing that would lead me to do in later life.

During this time I developed the next defence, which was the illegible handwriting – which is of course invaluable in a medical career. It is for some reason allowable to be unable to communicate due to poor handwriting but not due to poor spelling.

I discovered the typewriter during A levels, which interestingly helped with the spelling of simple words and if I switch off and type I make fewer mistakes and certainly do not make back to front letters. However, over the last few years, I have discovered that there is one thing better than a typewriter to improve spelling, and that is a good secretary!

Having dyslexia certainly shaped my life. Rather like the church mouse in the Somerset Maugham short story, where would I be now if I was normal? I may still have become a doctor, but I doubt whether I would have worked so hard or fought so aggressively to get to the top if I hadn't had so much to prove.

APPENDIX: EXAMPLES OF PARIS'S WORK

PARIS - 1st YEAR PRIMARY SCHOOL

Paris 15 March

I Went to the Cinema

and I saw Obelisk

PARIS - 2nd YEAR PRIMARY SCHOOL

The story of David and saul
I likeThe bit When The
shepherd boy Went to cut The
cloak in The cave instead of
Killing King saul / good

How North American Indians
live how there are pen Inbians but
there have corsant they still haven
canoes but they have motors on
them now

PARIS - 2/3rd YEAR PRIMARY SCHOOL

1. ti was a Magic TRUNK
   it cood Tfly and it was curious
2. The merchants was in side The
   TrunK
3. ti woud fly to a another
   couhtry
4. because when it flew it
   flew from the chimmy
5. because he cood get a hasty fall
6. in a foreign coutry
7. he concealed the Trunk under
   a heap
8. The traveller was wearing a
   dressing-gowh and slippers
9. decause evry body goes about
   wereing dressing-gown and slippe-
   arsi
10. a nurse with a baby
1 ervenchrs

Monday/19th March

<u>Exploring</u>

In London Jacob and Tom and Jahanell Went
shopping With Mum. First they Went to the
Supermarket. Shopping with Mum First they
Then We Went home We played a game. We Went
out We Went into somebody's house It w Was spooky
A monster shot out Tom stabbed him He was still alive
Jacob shoot him The monster Walsooded They Waked
into the house It was scary Suddenly Tom Was shot
We alked on Then four men came. Ust two took cover We
had a fight We fought as hard as W could After I reahsed
Where We shaould go. Next Jehan culleft and Jacod
Said the same thing got home.

PARIS - 4th YEAR PRIMARY SCHOOL

Friday 30th March 1984.
One day Jehan and Paris Whent oWt We
Went Down a cave We Saw a Dalek and
two Slug monsters. We Shot
them and more Came We Ran as Fast as We
could we got in a fight.
We took off. We Saw five duleks ships
Woflew then they Started shooting
We jumped to speed We destroyed
tow. We landed We had a fight then We
Went home, our Mums were Killed we
set a bout to destroy the daleks.
We Planed the bomb we destroyed the
daleks

two

110

At the centre of the earth
is the core. The inner core is
thought to be solid Scientists
have discovered this with the help of
a machine called a Seismograph
which can detect and record wave
movements deep in th earth. The
cor is very very hot.
It is not possible to dig down below
the earths crust to see the mantle and
the core.

PARIS - 5th YEAR PRIMARY SCHOOL
START OF THE JOINING UP OF THE HANDWRITING
6th YEAR - SAME AS THE 5th

Father william

"you are old, Father william",
the young man said,
"And your hkair has become very
wht white i
And yet you incessantly stand on
your head
Do you think at your age, it is right
right?"

Hebrew

Rosh Hashanah

In the Jewish calendar there is a period of ten days which are neither joyous or sad. This period of ten is known as the "ten days of Repentance" or the "ten days of Return". The ten days of Repentance begins the Jewish New year called Rosh Hashanah in Hebron, which occasions every year in September. Jews spend their time during the two days

PARIS - 1ST YEAR SECONDARY SCHOOL

3/10/87   <u>Arabic</u>

130,000,000 people speak this language. It started in the Middle East. Around the year 650, followers of mohammed conquered all of North Africa and southern Spain. Many Spanish words still show the influence of Arabic.

Hello Ehelen
How are you? Tina lebes
I'm fine, thanks ena lebes, shukran
goodbye bslema

112

PARIS - 2ND YEAR SECONDARY SCHOOL COMPUTER VERSION OF WRITING TEST
18-1-89
188 WORDS
2 SPELLING MISTAKES
1 WRONG WORD

THE ANIMALS REVOLT

It all started in a zoo, the cleaner there was a animal hater, he came to the zoo and went into the monkeys cage and poked, and hit them. The cleaner came as usual and when he went into the monkeys cage, and then out came all the monkeys hitting at the man. Then they escaped the man ran off out of the zoo. The monkeys went out of the zoo setting free all the animals, as the first of the animals came out. into the street people screamed and ran off down the road. The animals ran into the road hitting cars, climbing lamp posts and pushing down rubbish bins but no <u>teranchelers</u> got <u>louse</u>. The animals stampeded across the land and more and more animals got <u>louse</u> and the only one place was left not touched by the animals and that place was a small island off the coast of france. Because ⓐl the people of that Island were kind to animals, all the animals made those people <u>there</u> royal family and they lived in harmony. But all the animals were using people as pets.

THE END.

PARIS - 2ND YEAR SECONDARY SCHOOL
WRITING COMPARISON TEST
15-1-1989
150 WORDS IN 30 MINUTES
25 SPELLING MISTAKES

The End of they Earth

It was the year 1990 and the woulds arms race was at its peak and the leaders were USSR and USA those two countrys were at war there hade been no nucular wepons used but there had been much blood shed the fighting had stoped and there were nagos heations taking place but at prieslyprically 12.10 nagoreations had brocken down. and the presedend of of USSR had been taken prisoner and have dismandid all USSR nucular wepons. then after about 10 days the USSR agreed to the turms wharall the wepoas had been given to USA the USSR's presedent was reficed. and the USSR was taken over buy the USA and after the about a day a russan secret missile was lunched and the usa coal lunched a missile and bothe countrys were blown up and as they belw up it shook a weat spot in the earth and every countrey diserofied in to the center of the earth.

The End.

114

PARIS INNES
COMPUTER PERFORMANCE TEST RESULTS
21-10-89
374 WORDS IN 30 MINUTES
4 SPELLING MISTAKES
4 WRONG WORDS

THE DEMAND CLOCK

In my house there used to be a clock it was a hundred and
fifty years old and was hand painted and has two naked babys
on the sides   These babies were holding in there hands fire
touches   the old clock ticked away for years until one day
it stopped   We didn't take to the watch makers because it
would cost to much money to have it fixed   we are poor
family and we live in a drafty old house in the country
side   Any way when the clock stopped strange things started
happening to my family   at first we thought it was just bad
luck because it was just things going wrong first the car
wouldn't start and then the phone was dead but when we went
out to see the wires they had been cut   We all thought
something weird was going on so my dad got the gun out of
the cabinet and loaded it   We all stayed in the sitting
room but that was the worst mistake we could make because of
the clock but we didn't know that until it was to late   The
first of are family to get killed was my dad he was the
nearest to the clock   one of the doors of the clock opsned
and out came a hand and the hand grabbed my dad and choked
him till he died my little sister was the only one who saw
it happen but she is deaf and dumb and was two late two warn
my dad   My mother was the second to see my father and she
did not cry but she just grabbed the gun and pointed it all
around the room but she would have blown the clock up then
and there if she new that it had don it but she didn't and
I'm not sure it would have hurt it even if she did try   As
we sat there the day past quickly and we were all soon fast
asleep I don't know why but I felt really tied but now I
think it might have been the clock that made me tied   I was
aroused by my mother screaming she had one of the naked
babies on top of (end of test) my mother burning her back

115

PARIS INNES
WRITING PERFORMANCE TEST RESULTS
20-10-89
328 WORDS IN 30 MINUTES
39 SPELLING MISTAKES
10 WRONG WORDS

The Stelling of the croun jewls

On Christmas eve the crown jewls were stolen, I was an an inspector and this is my acount of the robery there were three drunken men out side the palace at 11:00 pm they proceed to nock out the gaud at the gate and scale the fence the alarm was aroused by the Security and gaurds were sent to aprehend the intruders so the gaurds arrived at the Sene they were shot and thrown in the moat. The three men went up to the Security gaurds rooms and shot every single one of them, the alarm had been raised and police were at the scene amediately the men carried on up towards the volt shooting gaurds as they went as they neared the main volt one of the men was shot by persuiving policemen. When they reached the volt they placed dinomite at the mouth and blow the volt open Killing two policemen the men then took the crown jewls and climbed to the top of the building were a microlite picked them up and flow them to a privet air port were they took a Air force jet and flew it to the jungle in africa. the jet was folowed there and was brought in, but the cremanles escaped into the jungle and are now being persued by the S.A.S. We have found out that the men Killed four gaurds in the prosess of the robery these men will be brought back deador alive.

<u>Singned</u> Inspector paris Innes

A newspaper head line.

The crown <u>jewles</u> Stolen by un know geng

A News flash we have discoverd <u>there</u> names
they are fred, bob and there Mum hitler. they were
dust bin men from <u>chealsea</u>.
the man whos <u>flow</u> the plane was prince charlse
and the one whos <u>flow</u> the <u>mikrowlite</u> was a
princess Die. Maggie <u>thacher</u> Said that
She <u>new</u> they couldn't be <u>trusted</u> and that she
Should be crowned queen of England.

WRITING PERFORMANCE TEST RESULTS
15-4-90
429 WORDS IN 30 MINUTES
(With 10 minute breaks after each 10 minutes- Cramp)
20 SPELLING MISTAKES
5 WRONG WORDS

The hover bike Race

It was a cold day and ~~Suddenly~~ Mikey sat on his hover bike waiting for the rest of his gang to show up. As he sat there he heard a raiving of hover bikes and around ~~came out~~ a corner came ~~last~~ it was Mikeys gangs rivals the gang started to race towards ~~the~~ Mikey and Mikey started up his bike and raced ~~after them~~ off. As he drove he could see the other gang behind ~~him~~ in the mirror ~~as~~ then suddenly they started catching up with him and soon they were right beside him they bashed him off the road and he fell off his bike. The other gang stopped there cycles and got off them they picked up Mikey and they beat him till he could not stand up then they road off after a well Mikeys gang came and picked up Mikey and took him to all to there hiding place ware Mikey told them what happaned and just as he finished Mikeys little brother burst in and told them there was going to be a big hover bike race and the prize was going to be a delux poolaros which was the fastest bike in the hole world. all of Mikeys gang entered and soon it came to the day of the race and they all lind up on the starting line Mickeys gang there rivels and lots of other competitos and then the lazer beam gate went up and they were off Mikey went straight in the lead followed closly by his rivals as they went round the first bend one of the other gang who was the leader when mame went blood suck over a big crang saver out of his bike and made knuckle go off the track and all the other competitos he started up the motor hover bike and was off again as they went round and round the track Mikey started to catch up and when he did there was no stopping him and soon he was just behind the leader and it was on the last lap. and he wouldn't let him past and as they were coming to the end of the race he pushed past the leader and just made it through to win

at the finish the blood got of his bike and went to hit Mickey when the police grabbed him from behind and pulled him to the floor and dragged him into the police car and took him away then the presentation was done and he was given the hover bike and he rode off into the sun set

This is a picture of the hover bike

PARIS INNES
COMPUTER PERFORMANCE TEST RESULTS
8-4-90
601 WORDS IN 30 MINUTES
3 SPELLING MISTAKES (1 word x 2)
9 WRONG WORDS (2 words x 3)

THE BIG WASH

The children were going to go to the ideal home centre in earls court. <u>There</u> mother was going to take them to see the biggest washing machine in the world. When they arrived they saw a sign saying this way to the biggest washing machine in the world when they arrived at the washing machine there was a guided tour of the machine and they would show it washing <u>cloths.</u> So the two children ran up to the old man who was selling tickets to the tour and they <u>brought</u> three and they all went on the tour. When it came to the showing of the working of the washing machine the children were to close to the edge of the place were they put all the <u>cloths</u> and they both fell in.

The two children went round and round until they saw a pipe way <u>were</u> they could get out and the two children went to the mouth of the pipe and swam in and at the other end of the pipe they saw a light so they swam for it and they soon came to the way out and they swam out and climbed out of the water when they climbed out they saw every one around them was gigantic and they were tiny so none of them saw them so they hid until the place was closed down so they could escape from the centre. When they did they found them selves in the street it was late and they <u>new</u> that <u>there</u> mother would be worried so they set off home.

They had been walking for hours when they saw a cat chasing them and they ran for <u>there</u> lives until they came to a small pipe which they could climb and when they got to the top they could see a man playing with toy remote control cars and so the little girl said to her brother "Bobby are you thinking what I am thinking" and Bobby said "yes" so the two children went down to <u>were</u> the man was playing with his remote control car and jumped on it when it passed them once they were inside they could make it so the remote control the man had did not control it any more and they could control it so <u>the</u> pulled some wires out and put some wires in different places and they were off at a great speed and the man who's car it was did not have a chance to stop them and they were off.

As they went along they saw people chasing them but they were just to fast for them to catch and as they were nearing the park near <u>were</u> they live the cars batteries ran out. When the car stopped the children jumped out and went into the park it was scary for the children and all the animals were ten times bigger than them and they kept hearing owls sounding and then children started to run as fast as the^y could but suddenly a great big claw grabbed them and then they were lifted off the ground and into the air and away from the ground. They were both taken to a nest were the children fell asleep.

The next morning the children were <u>woke</u> by an owl who could talk to them and it said that it would look after them and the children said they wanted to go home but the owl said that it would be hurt if they did not stay and it would have to kill them if they ran away.

PARIS INNES
COMPUTER PERFORMANCE TEST RESULTS
8-4-90
601 WORDS IN 30 MINUTES
3 SPELLING MISTAKES (1 word x 2)
9 WRONG WORDS (2 words x 3)

THE BIG WASH

The children were going to go to the ideal home
centre in earls court. There mother was going to take them
to see the biggest washing machine in the world. When they
arrived they saw a sign saying this way to the biggest
washing machine in the world when they arrived at the
washing machine there was a guided tour of the machine and
they would show it washing cloths. So the two children ran
up to the old man who was selling tickets to the tour and
they brought three and they all went on the tour. When it
came to the showing of the working of the washing machine
the children were to close to the edge of the place were
they put all the cloths and they both fell in.

The two children went round and round until they saw a
pipe way were they could get out and the two children went
to the mouth of the pipe and swam in and at the other end of
the pipe they saw a light so they swam for it and they soon
came to the way out and they swam out and climbed out of the
water when they climbed out they saw every one around them
was gigantic and they were tiny so none of them saw them so
they hid until the place was closed down so they could
escape from the centre. When they did they found them
selves in the street it was late and they new that there
mother would be worried so they set off home.

They had been walking for hours when they saw a cat
chasing them and they ran for there lives until they came to
a small pipe which they could climb and when they got to the
top they could see a man playing with toy remote control
cars and so the little girl said to her brother "Bobby are
you thinking what I am thinking" and Bobby said "yes" so the
two children went down to were the man was playing with his
remote control car and jumped on it when it passed them once
they were inside they could make it so the remote control
the man had did not control it any more and they could
control it so the pulled some wires out and put some wires
in different places and they were off at a great speed and
the man who's car it was did not have a chance to stop them
and they were off.

As they went along they saw people chasing them but
they were just to fast for them to catch and as they were
nearing the park near were they live the cars batteries ran
out. When the car stopped the children jumped out and went
into the park it was scary for the children and all the
animals were ten times bigger than them and they kept
hearing owls sounding and then children started to run as
fast as the^y could but suddenly a great big claw grabbed
them and then they were lifted off the ground and into the
air and away from the ground. They were both taken to a
nest were the children fell asleep.

The next morning the children were woke by an owl who could
talk to them and it said that it would look after them and
the children said they wanted to go home but the owl said
that it would be hurt if they did not stay and it would have
to kill them if they ran away.

ACKNOWLEDGEMENTS

We would like to thank the following people for their input, which helped make this book possible:

Rick Fuller, who realised that he was not stupid before the word dyslexia was commonplace. He was the first to tell us that typing seemed to help the problem. Rick is now one of the country's leading research doctors in the study of asthma.

The Dyslexia Teaching Association, Kensington, for their dedicated help in the basics and the comprehension of words.

Ray Sugden at Smith Corona for his help, and a product which has made it all possible.

Clare Harding, Paris's head of year, who enabled Paris to use the word processor in the school environment, and to all those at his school who have shown remarkable willingness and openness to new ideas that might help Paris. Many schools wouldn't have wanted the disruption.

Henry Rutkowski, for his patience with a computer illiterate, and especially for his help in getting our computer system working – no mean task, I can tell you, especially when it came to making all the bits 'talk to each other'.

Anne Hughes from Hughes PCS, for her help in making a hard disc portable more affordable, so that we could tackle the next stage of the dyslexic problem – maths!

Ian Jones of 'Central Maths' for taking the time to listen and for his dedicated help in solving our maths problems.

Dorothy, for helping us acquire the second PWP for Paris to use at home.

Francesca Cassavetti, for her illustration of the 'Computer Monster'.